D1563985

Antisocial Personality Disorder

A Practitioner's Guide to Comparative Treatments

Edited by

FREDERICK ROTGERS, PSYD, ABPP and
MICHAEL MANIACCI, PSYD

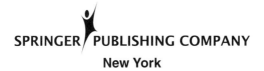

SPRINGER PUBLISHING COMPANY
New York

Springer Publishing Company, Inc.
11 West 42nd Street, 15th Floor
New York, NY 10036-8002

Acquisitions Editor: Sheri W. Sussman
Production Editor: Print Matters
Composition: Compset, Inc.

Library of Congress Cataloging-in-Publication Data

Antisocial personality disorder: a practitioner's guide to comparative treatments / [edited by]
    Frederick Rotgers, Michael Maniacci.
        p. ; cm. — (Springer series on comparative treatments for psychological disorders)
    Includes bibliographical references and index.
    ISBN 0-8261-5554-5 (hc)
        1. Antisocial personality disorder—Treatment. I. Rotgers, Frederick. II. Maniacci,
    Michael. III. Series.
        [DNLM: 1. Antisocial Personality Disorder—therapy. 2. Psychotherapy—methods. WM
    190 C7367 2005]
    RC555.C66 2005
    616.85'82—dc22

                                                                    2005054056

ISBN 0-8261-5554-5

06 07 08 09 10 5 4 3 2 1

Printed in the United States of America by Bang Printing

Contents

Contributors

Elissa M. Ball, MD, Institute for Forensic Psychiatry, Colorado Mental Health Institute. Pueblo, Colorado

Debra Benveniste, MA, MSW, Private Practice, Putnam, Connecticut

Katherine Anne Comtois, PhD, Department of Psychiatry and Behavioral Sciences, University of Washington, Seattle, Washington

Darwin Dorr, PhD, Wichita State University, Wichita, Kansas

Brian Eig, Department of Psychology, Philadelphia College of Osteopathic Medicine, Philadelphia, Pennsylvania

Carl Ake Farbring, MA, Swedish National Prison & Probation Administration, Stockholm, Sweden

Lars Forsberg, PhD, Department of Clinical Neuroscience, Section of Dependency Research, Karolinska Institute, Stockholm, Sweden

Arthur Freeman, EdD, Department of Psychology, University of St. Francis, Fort Wayne, Indiana

Joel I. D. Ginsburg, PhD, C. Psych, Psychologist, Correctional Service of Canada, Fenbrook Institution, Gravenhurst, Ontario, Canada

Robin A. McCann, PhD, Institute for Forensic Psychiatry, Colorado Mental Health Institute, Denver, Colorado

Sharon Morgillo Freeman, PhD, MSN, RN-CS, Indiana University Purdue University, Aboite Behavioral Health Services, Fort Wayne, Indiana

John M. Rathbun, MD, Aboite Behavioral Health Services, Fort Wayne, Indiana

Glenn D. Walters, PhD, Federal Correctional Institution, Schuylkill, Pennsylvania

CHAPTER 1

Antisocial Personality Disorder

An Introduction

Frederick Rotgers and Michael Maniacci

The therapy of patients with disorders of character or personality has been discussed in the clinical literature since the beginning of the recorded history of psychotherapy. Literature on the psychotherapeutic treatment of specific personality disorders has emerged more recently and is growing quickly. The main theoretical orientation in the psychotherapeutic literature on treatment of personality disorders has been psychoanalytic (e.g., Kernberg, 1975; Masterson, 1978; Reid, 1978). Psychoanalytic writers have produced a rich literature on treatment of these patients for more than 30 years.

More recently, cognitive behavioral therapists (e.g., Beck & Freeman, 1990; Young, 1994) have offered a cognitive behavioral treatment approach. Despite the literature in this area, there have been few opportunities for a comparison and integration of extant models. Very often, writers end up "preaching to the converted" in that those therapists who are psychodynamically oriented tend to read the psychodynamic literature just as cognitive and behavioral therapists stick to their own literature. Cross fertilization of approaches is thereby stymied.

Probably no single diagnostic group engenders as much concern, consternation, and fear among therapists as does Antisocial Personality Disorder (APD). This concern and attention stems from the fact that these patients usually require more time in treatment (when they come), more energy on the

1

part of the therapist (where the patient may offer very little to the therapeutic collaboration), and more time and attention from the care system (because of the chronicity of personality disorders), all without the same progress and gratification seen with many other patients. In fact, many therapists simply throw up their hands and claim that these individuals cannot be treated in psychotherapy. The patient diagnosed as having APD often ends up "clogging up" the legal and mental health systems, continually relapsing and given to extensive utilization of mental health treatment services with little positive change.

Given all of the difficulties in treating these patients, they still must be treated. The best model for treatment is debatable. Theorists often advocate the application of their etiologic, conceptual, philosophical, and treatment model, to the exclusion of other approaches. What has not, to this point, been explicated are the similarities and differences between various etiologic, conceptual, philosophical, and treatment models.

In this volume we attempt, in small measure, to provide a forum in which experts in prominent models of treatment for patients with APD all answer the same set of questions with respect to their treatment model, addressing both conceptual and technical aspects of the model. Authors were provided with a prototypical case study of a patient with APD to serve as the springboard for their answers.

Before we turn to the questions and a brief overview of APD, we need to state that this book is not intended to be a comprehensive survey of the treatment of APD. Rather, we have selected a number of prominent models of treatment that we believe span the psychodynamic, eclectic, and behavioral approaches to treating these patients. There are certainly other models available, and we do not intend to imply that these models are the only ones, nor that they are the most efficacious. We leave the latter judgment to outcome researchers, who are only recently beginning to examine outcomes specifically with APD.

STRUCTURE OF THE BOOK

In the remainder of this chapter we will present a brief overview of the construct of APD, with a focus on diagnostic considerations and several ongoing controversies regarding the construct of APD. We will not review the extant treatment outcome literature, for the primary reason that there is virtually no well-designed outcome research that focuses solely on APD outcomes. In fact, virtually all of the experimental treatment outcome research with these patients has occurred in the context of treatment of substance use disorders, a very common co-occurring set of disorders in patients with APD.

Following this overview, we will detail the questions our authors were asked to address with respect to the treatment of Frank J., whose case is presented in detail in chapter 2. The responses of our chapter authors follow. We will conclude in our final chapter with a summary and synthesis of the responses our authors provided. It is our hope that this discussion will stimulate not only development and enhancement of treatment for patients with APD, but that it will also provide impetus for outcome research on the treatments outlined.

OVERVIEW OF APD

In this section we will briefly review the history and construction of the concept of APD and the current criteria for its diagnosis, and we will describe some of the clinical features of the disorder that are most relevant for treatment. In addition, we will address two continuing controversies in the field regarding APD: the relationship of morality and criminality to APD, and the question of whether APD represents a qualitative or quantitative departure from normal personality functioning. Finally, we will examine the somewhat sparse outcome literature for the treatment of APD. Of necessity, this chapter will be less than comprehensive. For a more detailed discussion of these issues we would refer the reader to the excellent chapter on "Antisocial Personality Disorders: The Aggrandizing Pattern" in Millon and Davis's book *Disorders of Personality: DSM-IV and Beyond* (1996, pp. 429–469). Although written from a particular theoretical perspective, this chapter presents a detailed overview of the concept of APD and reviews in more detail the controversies we will only touch upon here.

The concept of APD is quite old, dating, in a surprisingly modern form, to Aristotle (Millon & Davis, 1996), whose description of the "unscrupulous man" is perhaps the earliest of this personality pattern. As the concept of APD evolved into the 18th and 19th centuries, it became increasingly linked with criminality and immoral behavior. This linkage persists today, and for some theorists (e.g. Millon & Davis) it represents a major problem in the current diagnostic system for APD. Specifically, the association of APD with criminal and immoral behavior needlessly limits the concept to those with criminal involvement or those whose behavior is considered immoral. Many theorists believe that this limitation results in the omission of many people whose personality functioning is clearly the same as that in persons who end up in the criminal justice system, but who never become so involved. It is believed that many people who show many of the behavioral characteristics of APD, but whose behavior is highly valued, and often encouraged, by society, are omitted from this diagnostic group because of this distinct focus on criminality and irresponsible behavior. Examples of these "omitted" personality types are, these theorists argue, to be found among highly successful businessmen, politicians, and leaders (Millon & Davis).

The question of the moral tone of the criteria for diagnosing APD is considered by some theorists to be at odds with recent attempts to make the diagnostic system (the DSM) more objective and research based. These theorists point to the elimination of the "disorder" homosexuality from the DSM in the late 20th century as an example of this trend (Millon & Davis, 1996).

Controversies such as these abound in the literature on APD. While making reference to them, we will not attempt to resolve these issues here. It is important to recognize these controversies, as they contribute to some degree, in our view, to some of the major issues in the treatment of APD. Specifically, the issue of countertransference, which many of our authors address explicitly in their chapters, carries with it the moral and ethical context in which the therapist was raised and trained. Much negative countertransference in treating patients with APD arises, in our view, from views of the morality and legality of behavior that are instilled developmentally in therapists by virtue of their having grown up in Western society.

The second controversy centers on whether or not APD represents a qualitatively different personality pattern or whether it is merely an extreme form of a cluster of personality traits and behaviors that are also found in individuals without personality disorders. This controversy also has an impact, in our view, on how therapists view and work with patients with APD. If APD is considered to be simply an extreme form of what is potentially a "normal" or non-pathological personality make-up, then treatment may hope to move the patient along the continuum toward the "normal" pole and lasting changes may be possible. However, if APD represents a qualitatively different form of personality and behavior (perhaps as the result of biological factors not found in patients who do not qualify for an APD diagnosis), then the task of treatment may become one of simply managing the symptoms and behaviors of APD, rather than producing a "cure."

The question of the dimensionality of APD is also seen in a persistent controversy surrounding the concept of "psychopathy" (Hare, Hart & Harpur, 1991). Many theorists believe that APD falls along a continuum of severity, with "psychopathy" representing the most impaired end of the continuum. The incidence of "psychopathy," conceived of as the most severe manifestation of APD, is lower than that of APD generally, but it is believed that these patients are among the most refractory to treatment. A continuing controversy in the field is whether patients who qualify for the designation of "psychopath" require qualitatively different treatment than do patients whose APD is less severe. There is also some controversy as to whether "psychopaths" are actually a different diagnostic group from patients diagnosed with APD, rather than representing a more severe form of a larger disorder.

With these controversies in mind, let us now turn to the criteria for diagnosing APD. These criteria themselves have evolved over the years and, while they are perhaps more useful in their current form than in historical forms, there is still room for refinement and improvement (Millon & Davis, 1996).

The DSM-IV-TR includes APD as one of what are termed "Cluster B" personality disorders. These disorders (the others in Cluster B include Borderline, Histrionic, and Narcissistic Personality Disorders) all share a tendency for patient behavior to be dramatic, emotional, or erratic (American Psychiatric Association [APA], 2000). As with all personality disorders, the traits and behaviors of APD must be more than transitory in order for the diagnosis to be made. Merely engaging in antisocial, criminal, or other behaviors associated with the diagnostic criteria is not sufficient to qualify a patient for a diagnosis of APD. The index behaviors and traits must be part of "enduring patterns of perceiving, relating to, and thinking about the environment and oneself that are exhibited in a wide range of social and personal contexts" (APA, p. 686). In order to qualify for a diagnosis of APD, the patient must have shown the characteristics of the disorder in many contexts and over a prolonged period of time. The DSM-IV-TR also requires that at least some of the behaviors that are central to APD be apparent prior to age 15 years in the form of evidence of Conduct Disorder. However the diagnosis of APD requires that the patient be at least 18 years old. The complete criteria for diagnosing APD are presented in Table 1.1.

The prevalence of APD is, fortunately, not high, with estimates in males clustering at about 3% and in women at 1% (APA, 2000). Although rare, it is clear that people with APD exact a toll in consequences to themselves and others far in excess of their numbers in the general population.

Persons who qualify for a diagnosis of APD also are highly likely to suffer from co-occurring disorders, most frequently a substance use disorder, although depression and anxiety disorders also occur in these patients. The most frequent co-occurring disorder is likely to be another personality disorder, however, particularly other Cluster B disorders (Millon & Davis, 1996). The presence of co-occurring psychopathology frequently complicates treatment, as will be seen in the case of Frank, to be presented later.

TABLE 1.1

DSM-IV-TR Diagnostic Criteria for Antisocial Personality Disorder

A. There is a pervasive pattern of disregard for and violation of the rights of others occurring since age 15 years, as indicated by three (or more) of the following:

1. failure to conform to social norms with respect to lawful behaviors as indicated by repeatedly performing acts that are grounds for arrest.

2. deceitfulness, as indicted by repeated lying, use of aliases, or conning others for personal profit or pleasure.

3. impulsivity or failure to plan ahead.

4. irritability and aggressiveness, as indicated by repeated physical fights or assaults.

5. reckless disregard to safety of self or others.

6. consistent irresponsibility, as indicated by repeated failure to sustain consistent work behavior or honor financial obligations.

7. lack of remorse, as indicated by being indifferent to or rationalizing having hurt, mistreated, or stolen from others.

B. The individual is at least age 18 years.

C. There is evidence of Conduct Disorder with onset before age 15 years.

D. The occurrence of antisocial behavior is not exclusively during the course of Schizophrenia or a Manic Episode.

From a more descriptive perspective, the DSM-IV-TR focuses on the essential feature of APD as being a "pervasive pattern of disregard for, and violation of, the rights of others . . . " (p. 701). Associated features include a lack of empathy, a callous and cynical worldview, and contempt for the feelings of others. These features are among those that have led to difficulty in the psychotherapeutic treatment of patients with APD, as it is believed that they are unable to form an adequate therapeutic relationship as a result.

Another clinical characteristic of patients with APD is an arrogant and inflated self image that is often manifested as being extremely opinionated and cocky. These patients are often glib, charming, and verbally facile. Many patients who meet criteria for an APD diagnosis are impulsive and have a history of aggressive or violent behavior. They are often irresponsible in relationships and with respect to obligations to others and exploit others to their own ends. Lawbreaking is common, although not universal, among these patients. Of note is a frequent lack of concern for themselves that mirrors their lack of empathy and concern for others. This results in a very high incidence of premature mortality among these patients. For example, Verona, Patrick, and Joiner (2001) found that signs of chronic antisocial behavior on the Psychopathy Checklist-Revised (Hare, 2003), a widely used measure of psychopathy and antisocial personality, were significantly correlated with prior suicide attempts in a sample of male prisoners.

From the perspective of treatment, the main concerns about working with patients with APD have to do with their lack of ability to empathize and "connect" with others on an emotional level, factors that make a solid working therapeutic relationship. Patients with APD have been found to terminate therapy earlier on average than other patients (Hilsenroth, Holdwick, Castlebury, & Blais, 1998). This issue takes prominence in the consideration of the case of Frank that our authors were asked to address. Also of concern from the perspective of treatment is the strong tendency toward impulsivity often seen in patients with APD. This may get in the way of generalizing gains made in session to their lives outside, as they often react to immediate contingencies without thinking through consequences. The possibility of anger and aggressive behaviors that are often manifest in an intimidating and aggressive stance toward others, including the therapist, is a frequent concern in working with these patients.

Treatment outcome research on APD specifically is largely lacking. In fact, our efforts to locate well-designed outcome studies specifically for APD met with no success. However, there is a body of research that suggests that when APD co-occurs with a variety of other Axis-I disorders, prognosis for treatment of those disorders is poorer (e.g. Compton, Cottler, Jacobs, Ben-Abdallah, & Spitznagel, 2003).

With this brief overview of APD in mind, we will now turn to the questions our authors were asked about the case of Frank, whose history will be presented in chapter 2.

QUESTIONS FOR AUTHORS

As with other volumes in the Comparative Treatments series, the questions our authors were asked about Frank are aimed at focusing their discussion of their treatments in a way that will allow side-by-side comparison with other approaches. In the interest of both space and interpretability, authors were asked to restrict the length of their answers. What follows are the specific instructions we provided to our authors.

Instructions for Authors:

We would like you to organize your response to this case in the following manner:

I. Please describe your treatment model in *no more than* 3–4 double-spaced pages.

II. What would you consider to be the clinical skills or attributes most essential to successful therapy in your approach? (1–2 pages).

III. It is important to the goals and mission of this volume that you answer *each* of the following questions regarding the enclosed case material. Please limit your response to each question to no more than two double-spaced pages (500 words).

1. What would be your therapeutic goals for this patient? What is the primary goal? What is the secondary goal? Please be as specific as possible.

2. What further information would you want to have to assist in structuring this patient's treatment? Are there specific assessment tools you would use (data to be collected)? What would be the rationale for using those tools?

3. What is your conceptualization of this patient's personality, behavior, affective state, and cognitions?

4. What potential pitfalls would you envision in this therapy? What would the difficulties be and what would you envision to be the source(s) of the difficulties?

5. To what level of coping, adaptation, or function would you see this patient reaching as an immediate result of therapy? What result would be long-term subsequent to the ending of the therapy (prognosis for adaptive change)?

6. What would be your timeline (duration) for therapy? What would be the frequency and duration of the sessions?

7. Are there specific or special techniques that you would implement in the therapy? What would they be?

8. Are there special cautions to be observed in working with this patient (e.g., danger to self or others, transference, countertransference)? Are there any particular resistances you would expect, and how would you deal with them?

9. Are there any areas that you would choose to avoid or not address with this patient? Why?

10. Is medication warranted for this patient? What effect would you hope/expect the medication to have?

11. What are the strengths of the patient that can be used in the therapy?

12. How would you address limits, boundaries, and limit-setting with this patient?

13. Would you want to involve significant others in the treatment? Would you use out-of-session work (homework) with this patient? What homework would you use?
14. What would be the issues to be addressed in termination? How would termination and relapse prevention be structured?
15. What do you see as the hoped-for mechanisms of change for this patient, in order of relative importance?

TREATMENT APPROACHES

To answer these questions we invited a group of authors whose theoretical positions range from avowedly psychodynamic, through more eclectic, to avowedly behavioral and cognitive behavioral.

The approaches we have included are: a psychodynamic approach based largely on object relations theory (Benveniste); an Adlerian approach (Maniacci); a biosocial learning approach based on Millon's broad conceptualization of personality disorders (Dorr); motivational interviewing, an avowedly Rogerian approach (Ginsburg, Farbring, & Forsberg); a largely eclectic approach based in Criminal Lifestyle theory (Walters); a more traditional cognitive behavioral approach (Freeman & Eig); and an approach based in Dialectical Behavior Therapy (Linehan, REF) which has been studied extensively for treatment of other personality disorders, specifically Borderline Personality Disorder (McCann, Comtois, & Ball).

We also enlisted a chapter exclusively on psychopharmacological approaches (Freeman & Rathbun). While still not to the point where medications can be used as the sole treatment for APD (if that will ever be the case), recent clinical literature has begun to include medications as a useful adjunct to psychotherapy with these patients. We therefore thought it important to provide readers with an overview of current psychopharmacological approaches to treating aspects of APD that can then be incorporated (and are incorporated by many of our chapter authors) into a broader spectrum treatment approach for these patients.

Let us now turn to our authors.

REFERENCES

American Psychiatric Association. (2000). *Diagnostic and statistical manual of mental disorders* (4th revised ed.). Washington, DC: Author.

Beck, A.T., & Freeman, A. (1990). *Cognitive therapy of personality disorders.* New York: Guilford.

Chessick. R.D. (1966). The psychotherapy of borderland patients. *American Journal of Psychotherapy, 20,* 600–614.

Hare, R.D. (2003). *Hare PCL-R technical manual* (2nd ed.). N. Tonawonda, NY: MHS.

Hare, R.D., Hart, S.D., & Harpur, T.J. (1991). Psychopathy and the DSM-IV criteria for antisocial personality disorder. *Journal of Abnormal Psychology, 100,* 391–398.

Hilsenroth, M.J., Holdwick, D.J., Castlebury, F.D., & Blais, M.A. (1998). The effects of DSM-IV cluster B personality disorder symptoms on the termination and continuation of psychotherapy. *Psychotherapy, 35,* 163–176.

Kernberg, O.F. (1975). Further contributions to the treatment of narcissistic personalities. *International Journal of Psycho-analysis, 55,* 215–247.

Lion, J.R. (1972). The role of depression in the treatment of aggressive personality disorders. *American Journal of Psychiatry, 129,* 347–249.

Millon, T., & Davis, R.D. (Eds.). (1996). *Disorders of personality: DSM-IV and beyond* (2nd Edition). New York: John Wiley.

Reid, W.H. (1978). The sadness of the psychopath. *American Journal of Psychotherapy, 32,* 496–509.

Verona, E., Patrick, C.J., & Joiner, T.E. (2001). Psychopathy, antisocial personality and suicide risk. *Journal of Abnormal Psychology, 110,* 462–470.

Young, J.E. (1994). *Cognitive therapy for personality disorders: A schema focused approach* (revised ed.). Sarasota, FL: Professional Resource Press.

CHAPTER 2

The Case of Frank

Arthur Freeman

Frank J. is a 48-year-old Caucasian male referred for evaluation and therapy via the court system as a result of drunk and disorderly charges placing him in violation of his parole. In his initial clinical assessment, he is described as about 6 ft 1 in. tall, fit looking with a muscular build, a deep tan, a scar on the bridge of his nose, and his hair stretched from one side of his head to cover his baldness. He was wearing an expensive Italian suit and shoes with stylishly coordinated silk shirt, tie, and kerchief. He was well-spoken, presenting to the interviewer with a demeanor of apparent warmth and familiarity mixed with an air of disdain that eluded tangible description. He appeared to use eye contact as a means of intimidating the interviewer rather than as a means of establishing rapport and enhancing communication and relatedness.

To obtain information from a broad range of individuals in Frank's world, releases to obtain information from Frank's wife and other close relatives were sought. They were only obtained following the intercession of Frank's parole officer due to Frank's resistance to signing release forms. Because of the rational concern expressed by Frank's wife regarding his well-being, combined with her understanding of the need for accurate assessment data, obtaining background information from potentially useful sources became a much less daunting task than expected.

BACKGROUND INFORMATION

Frank J. is the older of 2 brothers, 2 years older than his younger brother Jimmy. When he was age 7 years, his mother died of causes of which he was unsure. Both boys were raised primarily by their father, a career military man who was stationed periodically at Fort Riley, Kansas, while Frank and his brother lived at home in Pennsylvania under the supervision of various housemaids and relatives. The boys would often spend entire summers at their maternal grandfather's chicken farm in Delaware and again would have little adult supervision. Frank's father was described by Frank's maternal aunt as a heavy drinker who was often physically and verbally abusive toward his sons. His verbal interactions were typically characterized by a litany of insults, name-calling and put-downs, and without a word of encouragement or support he would often humiliate the boys in front of others as a form of punishment.

Frank's brother recalled an incident during a family gathering when he and his brother were aged 8 and 10 years where his father, while in a state of intoxication, became enraged at the boys because a football they were playing with accidentally bounced onto the picnic table. The boys were ordered to pull their pants down in front of all those present while their father proceeded to warm their bare hides with a wooden switch. Frank's brother remembers that Frank stood there stoically while he [the brother] was further derided for losing control of his bladder. He marveled at how he could hear an almost inaudible growl coming from Frank, while he himself would stand shaking and sobbing during these types of episodes. He finished by confiding: When I look back at my childhood, what I remember most about the holidays and family get-togethers is being berated and ridiculed by my drunken father.

Frank's maternal aunt became a fairly rich source of material regarding Frank's childhood experiences and presentation. She remarked that by the age of 3 years, he seemed different from the other children in the family. She found it most curious that he never seemed to cry or show signs of fear. She recalled that in contrast to his brother Jimmy, who wept openly during their mother's funeral, Frank showed no emotion at all. She added that she gradually came to the realization that Frank was not receptive to her attempts at expressing affection nor would he show any in return. She described that when he was little he was a real chore to baby-sit for as he seemed unable to stay focused on any one thing or activity for any length of time. He was so active and intense that she would be worn out just watching him. She recounted that when playing with other children, he was often aggressive and bullying and seemed to pay little regard to adult interventions. On many occasions the adults present would have to take turns physically restraining him. She noted that as he got older this energy more and more found its outlet in increasingly dangerous and risky behaviors. "I remember the time he dove off a 30 foot cliff into the bottom of a quarry apparently on a dare. He ended up in the emergency room unconscious and with a huge gash across his broken nose. He always seemed to have an assortment of bumps and bruises or a cast on a leg or an arm." In addition, he was always getting into fights, missing school, and running away from home.

She mused that he seemed to have a kind of secret life to which no one in the family was ever privy. At a loss to explain the many apparently expensive material items (clothing, shoes, wrist watches, etc.) she would find in Frank's room, she would nonetheless avoid questioning him for fear of a violent outburst. With some hesitation, she recounted an incident in which she overheard some of Jimmy's friends discussing an incident in which Frank, then 14 years old, was supposed to have been involved in a knife fight in which he stabbed an older boy following an argument at a craps game. "I never knew what to do when things like this would come up. Confronting Frank was always risky because of his temper and impulsiveness. I could never really trust that he wouldn't attack me physically . . . although he never did. Plus, I was only around the boys some of the time and couldn't really provide any consistent guidance or supervision. Telling Frank's dad about things was always risky because he would usually fly off the handle and likely brutalize the boys. It seemed like I was always stuck between a rock and a hard place where these boys were concerned."

Conversation with Frank's brother Jimmy revealed a pattern of behavior in Frank that began to manifest itself when Frank was about 7 years of age. "I'll never forget the time I saw him douse a cat with gasoline and set it on fire. He just stood there laughing as the thing howled. I got sick to my stomach and ran home horrified. Another time he caught a frog at the pond on my grandfather's chicken farm. He then proceeded to cut its back legs off and stuffed its mouth with fire crackers and blew it up." Jimmy recalled the time that Frank took him to see the tree house he had built in the woods adjacent to their grandfather's farm. "He had lain several 2 by 6 inch boards from one large branch to another and fastened them with nails. This thing seemed like it was 50 feet up in the air. There were no branches low to the ground so you needed a tall ladder just to reach the large branches beneath it. I was always a little afraid of heights but he managed to dare me into climbing up there. Once I got up there and looked down, I froze in panic. Frank began pushing me toward the edge. I started to scream but couldn't move because it was like I was paralyzed. When he got me to the edge he started pushing me and then grabbing me, pushing me and grabbing me. All the while I'm screaming and bawling, he's laughing and calling me chicken. Finally, he lets go of me and climbs down to the ground. Next thing I know, he takes the ladder and walks off into woods with it. I yelled and yelled for him to put the ladder back but he just kept going. I remember staying up there for what must have been 3 or 4 hours until it started getting dark. My fear of being stuck up there became greater than my fear of heights and so I decided to take my chances jumping from the lowest branch. It was still too high and I ended up breaking my wrist. Frank threatened to kill me if I told anybody what happened."

According to Jimmy, he and Frank began drinking alcohol in their early teens. "There was always a supply of whiskey in the house and my father could never keep track of how much he had or how much he drank. When we were younger he used to give us beer and get us drunk for his own amusement." According to Jimmy, Frank was binge-drinking on weekends by age 16 years. During his last 2 years of high school he was suspended several times for drinking or being drunk during school hours. In spite of all the suspensions and truancy Frank always found ways to get passing grades.

Murph, an old high school acquaintance and close friend of Jimmy, Frank's brother, described Frank as "bold, fearless, and clever and he was always the toughest kid in the neighborhood." According to Murph, "Frank seemed to develop this uncanny streetwise savvy with an ability to read and know people from Jump Street. He could sell ice to Eskimos and always knew how to push people's buttons even if he never met them before. In class he would always terrorize the substitute teachers, especially the younger female teachers. He would first turn on the charm and then he would begin to get personal."

Murph recounted that in one instance, after complementing one of the female substitutes on some information she had presented to the class and making it seem as if he was really interested, Frank began to ask insulting questions about her clothes disguised as concern over her fashion awareness. He would then begin to weave in remarks about her physical features so subtly that it took her a while to realize that she had been made the subject of public ridicule. With this sudden awareness that she been duped and betrayed, she began to lose her concentration, turned beet red, and walked out of the room shaking like a leaf. Frank was apparently left to bask in his latest triumph, showing no concern for the pain he had just caused another human being.

According to Murph, this kind of interaction was typical of most of Frank's interactions with others. While he had many acquaintances and admirers, he had no close friends and would appear to humiliate and alienate those who attempted to get close to him. According to Murph, one of Frank's classmates had begun to look upon Frank as kind of a hero. "It got to a point where Frank was using this kid as his personal servant. He would get Frank's lunch, carry his books, do Frank's homework, anything Frank wanted. On the other hand, Frank never seemed to miss an opportunity to humiliate this kid whenever there was a crowd to show off in front of. As this relationship continued, Frank got more and more abusive toward the kid. Once Frank had a couple of guys help him tie the kid up and lock him in the trunk of his car and they all got drunk and went joy-riding. The other two guys involved started getting worried about the kid and told Frank that the joke had gone on long enough. Frank then stopped the car and left the two of them out in the middle of nowhere and took off. I was never sure what happened after that, but I know the kid ended up in the hospital all battered and bruised and dehydrated. He never told the truth about what happened."

Upon graduating from high school, Frank immediately joined the Marine Corps. He went to flight school and became a helicopter pilot in the Viet Nam war. His wife, Jennifer, related that Frank received three letters of commendation for bravery in the face of enemy fire while serving two tours of duty and eventually achieved the rank of Lieutenant. Photographs of Frank, taken during his years in the service, suggested to Jennifer that Frank had found a sense of meaning and purpose in his role as a soldier. "In just about all of the pictures, he has a smile on his face and a look in his eyes that I have rarely seen since I've known him. There is a sense of pride and contentment showing on his face, in his body language, and in the way he wears his uniform." In contrast to these impressions, Jennifer recounted how Frank would downplay his wartime experiences and achievements and once shocked her by suggesting how fortunate he was to actually get paid for killing a bunch of "gooks." To further confound the impressions she had gleaned from the photographs, she had overheard on a couple of occasions acquaintances and family members making reference to Frank's almost being court marshaled for his alleged involvement in gambling and black market operations involving stolen military supplies. "I always had great difficulty reconciling these stories with my feelings about Frank and found it easy to dismiss them as the product of jealousy."

After receiving an honorable discharge from the military, Frank returned to the family home in Pennsylvania. Less than 24 hours had elapsed when Frank got into a fistfight with his brother and attempted to run Jimmy over with his father's Chevrolet. "I really think the son-of-a-bitch would have run me over if I hadn't jumped real quick. That was the last anybody heard from him for a couple of years. We got wind from my wife's sister that he showed up at her place in Beverly Hills, borrowed about two grand from her and then disappeared."

According to records obtained from the criminal justice system, Frank joined the Los Angeles Police Department about 8 months after his arrival in

California. After 2 years on the force, he was dismissed following incidents of suspected brutality, taking bribes, and a series of disciplinary actions related to drinking while on duty. In one instance, Frank was accused of forcing a man he had stopped on suspicion of drug dealing to drop his pants and then inserting the barrel of his pistol into the suspected perpetrator's rectum. Frank's supervisor in those days, now a retired police captain, recalled that Frank always seemed to have a chip on his shoulder when it came to dealing with his superiors. "Any time you gave this guy a direct order, he'd give you this cold, icy stare like he wanted to slit your throat. If you confronted him about his reaction he'd try to make it seem as if you were losing touch with reality. When all these complaints and accusations started coming in, he developed this conspiracy theory, which he tried to sell to some of his fellow officers. He was blaming everybody from the police chief on down as being out to get him. At one point, he even had me half convinced that something like that was going on." Regarding the actual dismissal, the captain recalled that Frank probably thought that something really serious was about to come down and he seemed like the kind of guy who knew how to stay one step ahead of trouble. Because of his suspected drinking problem, Frank was offered the option of entering a treatment program as a condition of remaining on the force. He rejected this out of hand and quickly agreed to a dismissal.

Not long after this, Frank became part owner of a car dealership specializing in the sale of used foreign sports cars. According to Frank's parole officer, records suggested that Frank's business may have been based partly on the sale of both stolen and defective vehicles. Complaints that some of the vehicles sold were missing serial numbers sparked further investigation. Although he vehemently denied culpability, Frank was accused of selling stolen vehicles, vehicles with defective parts, and vehicles with apparent tampering of the odometer. Although none of these charges resulted in convictions, Frank eventually was investigated by the IRS and charged with income tax evasion. He spent almost 2 years in hiding, living in a brick addition he had built adjacent to his cousin Nick's restaurant in Sonora, New Mexico.

A telephone interview with Nick revealed that Frank had made several promises to Nick and his wife in exchange for his new living accommodations. "We all agreed that he would help out with the cooking, cleaning, and dish washing. It didn't take long for us to realize that Frank considered such work well beneath him. He always had some kind of excuse for why he couldn't help out. He would be gone for days at a time and we'd have no idea of his whereabouts. I finally got tired of hinting around and gave him an ultimatum of helping out, paying rent, or leaving. Since I had paid for the materials and did most of the work on the addition myself, I definitely felt like I was being used. As a result of the ultimatum, Frank and I got into a heated argument, during which blows were exchanged followed by Frank's storming out of the restaurant. A few days later, I noticed that all of his things were gone so I figured that that was all we would hear of Frank. The next morning as my wife was preparing to open the kitchen, I heard this loud shrill of horror coming from the kitchen area. I rushed downstairs to find Jan standing frozen and trembling. There, sitting inside one of the cabinets, was one of the largest diamond back rattlesnakes I have ever seen. We called the police but decided not to pursue charges."

Frank eventually surrendered to authorities and spent 3 years in jail followed by 5 years probation for income tax evasion. Three years after his release from prison, at the age of 46 years, Frank began dating an attractive young woman (16 years his junior) whom he married 10 months later. His wife, Jennifer, described the first year of their relationship as "the most exciting year of my life. He was just so spontaneous and full of energy. His charm and good looks just swept me off my feet. Being with him was just so exhilarating! At the drop of a hat he would tell me to grab some things, 'we're going on a trip,' and off we'd go to Las Vegas or Acapulco. Twice in that year he surprised me with plane tickets to Europe—we spent 3 days in Switzerland and 2 months later a week in Rome. We'd spend a lot of time in nightclubs where Frank would introduce me to various business associates. I became a little concerned with how much he drank but he never seemed to get really drunk or out of control. Frank certainly didn't seem to have the kind of problem with alcohol that my father had."

Jennifer recalled that shortly after she agreed to marry Frank, "it suddenly dawned on me that I really didn't know anything about him. He'd talk some about his relatives, but never seemed to have any contact with them. All I knew about his employment was that he was in real estate and land development and seemed to conduct most of his business by phone. He had an office in the home with little else in it but a desk, a phone, and stacks of Racing Forms. Frank seemed to get calls at all times of the day and night on his office phone. I could never quite understand why he insisted on keeping most of those business calls so private."

A number of incidents during the first year of the marriage caused Jennifer increasing concern. She found that she had to be extremely careful about how she acted around other men in social situations. "If I laughed too hard at one of their jokes, if I spent too much time talking with any one of them in particular, or if I seemed to contradict what Frank was saying, he would clobber me with silence the rest of the night. It might be days before I'd find out what was really bothering him."

Frank's drinking and occasional aggressive behavior also became an area of increasing concern for Jennifer. "On one occasion we were having dinner in the bar area of a restaurant. Frank had already had four Jack Daniels on the rocks before our dinner arrived. Soon after we had finished eating, Frank got into an argument with a patron at the bar. Frank suddenly got out of his chair and grabbed the man by the neck, threatening to kill him. I'll never forget the look on his face or the chilling sound of his voice as he said 'Either shut up or you're dead.' The man involved seemed as shocked and terrified as I was and quickly backed off and left the bar. This was the first time in the 13 months we were together that I'd seen this side of Frank and I just sat there in disbelief. Frank made some reference to the guy deserving what he got and more and quickly changed the subject. He showed absolutely no awareness of or concern over the effect the incident had on me."

Jennifer related that after this incident she had become increasingly aware of Frank's mood swings and irritability. "There were times when he would blow up at me for no apparent reason. What I found most upsetting though were the subsequent silent treatments that sometimes lasted for days, Then for some unknown reason he would just resume talking to me as if nothing had happened. Then there was the time he found out that I had been seen having lunch with a man who was an old friend of my family. He questioned and harangued me about this for almost a week. Nothing I said seemed to matter, as if he was just looking for an excuse to punish me. The episode ended with Frank's pulverizing my entire collection of Chinese tea cups, probably the only material possessions that had any real meaning to me. Frank knew this, and I was absolutely devastated that he could behave in such a cruel manner toward me. He never once apologized and he made it clear to me that I deserved it. After this episode, I made up my mind that either he or both of us needed some help."

According to Jennifer, the nature of Frank's employment had become increasingly unclear to her. She had trouble understanding why business calls kept coming in at all hours of the day and night. She knew that Frank was partners in a land development company and she had been to his place of business a couple of times earlier in their relationship. She again grew suspicious after calling Frank's office and learning that the phone had been disconnected. Frank's response to her query was that his secretary must have somehow forgotten to pay the bill.

"The clincher came when I drove up there to see him and found the door padlocked and all of the business signs gone. I remember feeling this intense mixture of anger and fear. Although I was livid that he would keep something like this from me, I was very much afraid of confronting him about it. At this point I kind of panicked and decided that I needed to get away from Frank for a while." Jennifer decided to stay with a friend who lived about 20 miles away until she could sort out what to do. "It took Frank 3 days to locate me by phone. When I explained my reason for leaving, he apologized profusely, claiming that it was just a miscommunication that he would further explain when I got home." Frank explained to Jennifer that his partner had gotten involved in some kind of land development swindle which Frank insisted he had no knowledge of or part in. As a result of the trouble, he and his partner decided that it was best to close down operations at least for the time being. Frank also acknowledged that he had begun taking a few bets from some race track junkies to try and keep their heads above water financially.

Shortly after this, an incident at a bar resulted in Frank's being charged with drunk and disorderly and aggravated assault. This meant that Frank was now in violation of parole. Through the insistence of his parole officer and at the behest of his wife, Frank reluctantly agreed to see a therapist for counseling.

INITIAL ASSESSMENT

Frank was initially very pleasant and charming with the female assessment interviewer, complimenting her on her dress and appearance, When questioned as to the reasons for coming to the interview, Frank instantly became irritated, stating: "I've been on my own all of my life. I've never needed any help from anybody. How much money do you make anyway? Why are you in this business? Why don't you make believe you have a life of your own?" The assessment interviewer got the impression that Frank had begun sizing her up immediately and very quickly figured out which buttons to push. Although shaken by this initial interaction, she proceeded to complete the interview.

In response to questions related to the issue of alcohol abuse, Frank laughed at the question and vehemently denied the problem. He described himself as a two-fisted drinker, a lover of life, and always in control of any situation in which he found himself. Frank bristled at the notion that alcohol had any control over him.

In discussing his rather labyrinthine employment history, Frank made references to all the poor slobs who work 9 to 5 jobs for other people, referring to these folks as suckers and slaves. Frank remained essentially uncooperative throughout the remainder of the interview process.

Combining her observations with historical data and the results of psychological testing, the following DSM IV diagnoses were made:

Axis I: 305.00 Alcohol Abuse
Axis II: 301.7 Antisocial Personality Disorder

Assessment data, including the results of both the Rorschach and MMPI, were used to rule out any history or indication of manic episodes or schizophrenia.

CHAPTER 3

A Psychodynamic Approach

Debra Benveniste

I. Please describe your treatment model.

My treatment model derives from both psychodynamic and trauma theory. Psychodynamic theories that are applied, e.g., attachment (see Bowlby, 1982; Crittendon, 1995), relational (see Mitchell, 1988; Russell, 1998), and object relations (see Buckley, 1986; Fairbairn, 1952), teach that human development, both normal and pathological, occurs within the context of relationships with significant others. Affect (feelings) and behavior are both attachment-driven. The internal structures of the personality are formed as a result of interaction in attachment-based relationships." If there is adequate nurturing in the form of the holding environment (Winnicott, 1972), then the person can develop into a functioning adult. Freud's succinct but encompassing statement of what defines a functioning adult is the ability to love and to work. If nurturing is inadequate, neglectful, or outright abusive, the personality that is forming must contort itself to accommodate this inadequate sustenance and normal development is derailed."

Trauma theory (see Allen, 2001; Van der Kolk, 1989) studies how the derailment process occurs.

"This character organization can be described from the perspective of brain function. Memories of traumatic experiences are stored in the more primitive parts of the brain, not accessible to the frontal cortex which houses the complex thinking processes. Due to the traumatic nature of the event when experienced, perceptions and the accompanying affects were fragmented and stored as such. Isolated memory fragments and affects seem to appear to the person at random" (Allen, 2001).

If we accept the concept that a personality forms around these discon-nected blips of experience and emotion, the result of a traumatic experience easily could be a personality disorder. This person does not have conscious access to the affects of traumatic memories. When asked to talk about a trau-matic event, there is no affect apparent in the presentation, yet when uncon-sciously triggered, affects appear and are overwhelmingly terrifying. Because they are not processed in the frontal cortex, they are also not anchored in time. All affects and memory fragments feel as if they are occurring in the present but simultaneously as if they have always been there. Additionally, defenses used to repress traumatic events prevent the person from relating in a genuine and spontaneous way.

Just as dysfunction is produced from inadequate relationships, this model theorizes that healing is derived from adequate attachments. The therapeutic· relationship is carefully structured to promote both healing from relationship-based traumas and personality change, defined as improvement in affect tolerance and ego functions. Affect tolerance is the ability to expe-rience feelings appropriate to the given situation, label them correctly, and communicate them effectively, such that the level of affect does not over-whelm the ego. The ego is the conscious part of the personality whose pri-mary function is regulatory. The superego, the part of the personality which develops moral values and produces guilt, is also a critical focal point in this case. Ego functions which are the most damaged or undeveloped in people with severe character pathology are: affect management (the ability to cope with a variety of feelings on a continuum of intensity), impulse control, judg-ment, object relations (the ability to establish and maintain genuine, mutual, and intimate relationships), and the functioning of the superego (Bellak, Hurvich, & Gediman, 1973).

Frank J. is a man whose experience in significant relationships began with early maternal loss, the most psychically destructive event in life. Chil-dren experience annihilation anxiety when the parent who safeguards their lives is suddenly and permanently gone. It is unclear what the nature of Frank's relationships with his parents were prior to his mother's death. Ad-ditionally, the cause of her death is unknown to Frank (and to the evaluator). Frank's father abandoned any parental role toward his sons after his wife's death (if in fact he had any prior) and was quite sadistic in his continual and public abuse and humiliation of his sons. Frank was unable to establish con-sistent attachments to any of the parental surrogates available to him. (Note the adults enabling Frank's father's abuse and his maternal aunt's abandon-ment of a parental role when she avoided questioning Frank for fear of a violent outburst.) Frank's level of distress in childhood was overwhelming at the very time that he would normally be developing ego functions which would help him both tolerate that distress and develop relationships with others that would help him contain it and feel safe (Allen, 2001).

Frank's childhood experience of relating with people is that they die and abandon him, are abusive and dangerous, or are neutral toward him but completely ineffectual at keeping him safe. These patterns become relational templates. Frank responds in relationships as if they are the only possible outcomes. He is continually guarding against the intense emotional danger that these perceived eventualities represent. This is the stance from which Frank approaches his therapist. The challenge (and goal) of this therapy is to establish a genuine empathic connection with Frank such that his traumas and structural defects of personality can be accessed and addressed.

From a traditional psychoanalytic point of view, treatment focuses on interpreting transference. Transference is an unconscious means with which the client experiences the therapist based on his attachment patterns from the past. For example, if the client's parents humiliated him during child-hood, he will experience the therapist as humiliating him in the present. In-terpretation, articulating the dynamics of these interactions, brings forward the working-through process. The client learns through this process that the dynamics do not apply in the therapeutic relationship, thus changing the client's personality structure to permit a distinction between past and present and to expand the client's relational templates. The focus of relational thera-pists is on the transference-countertransference interplay within the therapy relationship. The therapist's affective responses to the client and how they are communicated are considered as integral to the client's improvement and healing as the client's communications to the therapist. This model of therapy is more suited to traumatized clients' needs, as the traditional approach pro-duces too much anxiety (Bromberg, 1998).

Transference feelings are expressed verbally except in the case of the severely traumatized and characterologically impaired client who is unable to express in words the depth of his damage and despair or the terror at the prospect of doing so (Bromberg, 1998). Instead, affects are communi-cated unconsciously through behavior, known as the repetition compulsion. The client unconsciously creates conditions within the therapy whereby the therapist experiences these affects as his or her own (see question 15). Inter-pretation with this population cannot occur until affects are conscious. And affects cannot be experienced consciously until it is safe to do so. In our case, Frank would have to be ready to risk that the therapist will not abandon or torture him, or be present but ineffectual. How the affects are contained by the therapist, processed with the client, and ultimately returned to him comprise the basic components of this model of therapy.

II. What would you consider to be the clinical skills or attributes most essential to successful therapy in your approach?

The most essential skill in approaching this client from a psychodynamic framework is the therapist's use of an observing ego (Casement, 1985). The observing ego is that part of the therapist's mind that observes the interaction between him or herself and the client. It floats freely and carefully observes the client's words, facial expressions, tone, change of subjects, and body language. It also observes the same aspects in the therapist and his or her own thoughts and feelings about what is being communicated. This skill is of paramount importance in any psychodynamic therapy but particularly so with a client who has severe deficits in affect tolerance and verbal communication.

The most essential aspect of the observing ego in treating Frank is the ability to experience and interpret one's countertransference reactions. They are the source of understanding Frank's affects, as Frank can only communicate them through the use of projection. For example, Frank began the assessment interview by "complimenting her (the interviewer) on her dress and appearance." There is no mention of the interviewer's response to these comments; however, the clinical information indicates that this behavior begins a pattern for Frank of humiliating female authority figures. Later in the assessment, the interviewer became aware that Frank had been looking for and found "her buttons."

Compliments generally indicate boundary problems, veiled aggression, and the client's need to be seductive; to either disarm or distract the therapist. These issues relate to control and humiliation. Frank would not have been able to verbalize how central these issues are to his personality structure or his current difficulties. But if the interviewer had been observing her responses to Frank's "compliments," she might have expected the forthcoming narcissistic attack and then been prepared to look for its sources. Tolerance for intense, disturbing affects, one's own as well as the client's, is essential in this work (Coen, 2002).

Sociopathic people implicitly believe that there are few ways with which human beings relate: through intimidation, competition, use of scams, or through a mutual use pact ("you scratch my back and I'll scratch yours"). They are often quite controlling interpersonally and are known for their continual rule breaking. These traits are experienced by the client as ego syntonic; an asset, not a problem. Hedges (2000) refers to this as an organizing transference, a means with which the client maintains safety in emotional distance. Yet in their life circumstances, sociopaths are often controlled by others. Therapists are forced into the role of authority figure with this client population while conversely being barraged by feelings of helplessness engendered by the chronic lying and demanding behaviors. It is important for the therapist to be able to provide a balance for these interpersonal deficits despite the challenging nature of this task. Acceptance of how the client perceives and experiences others including the therapist is necessary, no matter how repellant those views may be. The therapist must engage in a genuine, respectful, and non-exploitative manner in order to provide a corrective experiential model for Frank and to establish a therapeutic alliance. Patience and tenacity are useful traits. A sense of humor helps, too.

1. What would be your therapeutic goals for this patient? What is the primary goal? The secondary goal?

The primary therapeutic goal in work with this patient is to establish a therapeutic relationship. The second is to contain destructive behavior. There are many other equally important goals to attain here but they are all predicated on the successful accomplishment of these two.

A successful therapeutic relationship is in place when the client feels accepted, understood, and respected by the therapist; trusts that the therapist has his best interests at heart; and feels that he can be open about himself without being judged. Psychodynamic therapy uses the therapeutic relationship as its method of intervention and healing, so that if there is no working alliance, no work can be done. Clients with antisocial personality disorder are arguably the most difficult to engage therapeutically, so this primary goal is also the most difficult to realize.

If no working relationship is established, one of three things will likely happen. The first is that Frank will infuriate the therapist to such a degree that he or she will refuse to continue to work with him (abandonment). The second scenario is that Frank will use his narcissistic skills to appear to take in and learn what is being presented to him. In this way, he will convince the therapist of his progress; he can continue to act out in the community; and, depending upon how good he is at it, he might even be able to convince the therapist to advocate for him when he inevitably gets in trouble (neutral but ineffectual). The third scenario is that Frank will succeed in humiliating and upsetting the therapist but he or she will feel it necessary to continue to work with him. In this case, there are either endless power struggles which Frank relies on to maintain distance or the therapist will take the victim role allowing Frank the sadistic stance (abusive). These situations reinforce the relational templates of Frank's early attachments.

A therapeutic relationship is not fully established until an initial treatment plan is developed. This plan is a product of both client and therapist, so Frank's treatment goals must be represented here as well. Once established, it is possible to intervene to reduce Frank's acting out behavior. From a psychodynamic point of view, the relationship itself will begin this process. The purpose of acting out is to discharge intolerable affect. The treatment model indicates that Frank's acting-out behavior derives primarily from a weak ego (impulsivity) and the need to reduce humiliation, feel in control, and keep people at a distance. If Frank had a relationship with his therapist where he felt accepted, his need to reduce humiliation would subsequently decrease. If he felt respected by his therapist, he would feel more in control to be able to set therapeutic distance where he needed. Frank would then have less need for his off-putting behavior as he would have a more appropriate way in which to set distance. His impulses would begin to be contained by this reduction in anxiety and defensiveness. As Frank's behavior and mood improved, his capacity to inhibit his impulses and reduce destructive acting-out would strengthen.

2. What further information would you want to have to assist in structuring this patient's treatment? Are there specific assessment tools you would use (data to be collected)? What would be the rationale for using those tools?

This is an interesting question, as the case information presented is necessary for each of us to formulate a treatment approach. However, were this an actual client presenting himself in my office, I would be operating with far less information from external sources and would not seek any more other than from Frank himself.

First, I would speak with Frank's parole officer to find out what precipitated the referral. I would want to know Frank's criminal record. Most importantly, I would want the parole officer's assessment of whether Frank posed a physical threat to me. I maintain a solo practice so my first concern with a client with Frank's background is my safety. Other than that, I would not have pressured Frank to sign further releases. I would have taken a history from him as I would from any client, but most likely in an informal manner over the course of several sessions. I would prioritize establishing a working relationship above gathering data.

Many therapists who treat clients with antisocial personality disorder become frustrated with the chronic lying, take it personally, and reject outright the information being presented. In fact, in this case, the only information gleaned directly from Frank comes from his defended/provocative comments about his coming to counseling, his drinking, and his employment history. In how many other cases would the client's own report be so thoroughly discounted?

No client, no matter how healthy, tells "the truth" during an initial assessment. Clients share the sources of their distress but their impaired capacities which bring them to treatment limit what they are able to perceive, experience, and articulate. They also want to look good. The difference with antisocial clients is that they deliberately lie. Rejection of a client's statements due to a determination that it is a lie is an unfortunate assessment technique. Two vital pieces of information can be discovered from a lie: the underlying wish and the direction in which the client is attempting to manipulate the therapist's impression of him. If I accept what he says, Frank will let his defenses down (perhaps initially because he thinks I am stupid for believing him). I would be establishing a therapeutic alliance while simultaneously obtaining more information. A stance of evenly suspended attention (Moore & Fine, 1990) helps to avoid over-reliance on the categorization of truth versus falsehood. Clients' communications are far too complex to be reduced in such a simplistic manner, particularly when the client is so unable to communicate directly.

That said, there are several specific pieces of information which I would want to know: Frank's level of psychopathy (see question 4), his history of relationships with women prior to age 46 years, the cause of his mother's death, and the length of his parole. I do not use ordinary assessment tools because as a social worker I would have to refer clients to a psychologist for testing. I only do so when I suspect significant neurological impairment, which I do not in this case.

3. What is your conceptualization of this patient's personality, behavior, affective state, and cognitions?

The two main events which shaped Frank's personality are his mother's death and the ongoing abuse and neglect he suffered from his primary caretakers. As a child, Frank coped with this onslaught by "asking with fists: disclaiming need through strategies of aggressive control" (Culow, 2001 p. 141). Shengold (1989) describes traumatization to this degree in a child as causing a "terrible and terrifying combination of helplessness and rage—unbearable feelings that must be suppressed for the victim to survive" (p. 2). Van der Kolk (1989) states that abused men and boys identify with the aggressor and later victimize others. Frank identifies with the aggressor to protect his connection with his father and distance himself from his childhood feelings (Fairbairn, 1992). The formation of the superego which emerges during the latency stage, ages 6–10 years, would have been completely derailed by Frank's mother's death. Psychopathic behavior was first noted in him at age 7 years. Fairbairn states that when relationships with primary caretakers are inadequate, children engage in sadism (relationship with an internalized object) as a substitute for "natural emotional relationships which have broken down." Crittendon (1995) describes aspects of the developing character of what she terms "coercive children" which apply to Frank, including a lack of ability to identify and label feelings, extreme and rapid mood shifts, and an inability to achieve sufficient mental distance for the integration of cognitive and affective integration. She states that coercive children can be expected to show disorders of behavior which emphasize angry/threatening/fearless acting-out that draw attention to themselves, and disorders of thought which emphasize one's own or other's hostility, power, and control that both deflect responsibility away from themselves and also suggest that there are few causal relations.

As a teenager, Frank began to rely on trauma-based coping strategies of dissociation, numbing, and substance abuse. As the developmental tasks of each age Frank reached became increasingly complex, he fell further behind. Criminal behavior met several needs for him. Breaking the law is an effective means with which to discharge rage and to "get high." And getting away with it reinforces a feeling of accomplishment.

Little information about Frank's relationships with women is available. From the perspective of a 7-year-old, Frank would conclude that he lost his mother because he is fundamentally unlovable, that he didn't deserve to keep her. Intimate relationships with women would elicit this unconscious belief that women will ultimately reject and abandon him

Frank exhibits some ego strength in the form of maintaining a marriage, some level of employment, and some control of his alcoholism. However, the amount of unprocessable affect continuously overloads his ego. Frank then becomes paranoid and his thought process paralyzed. Impulsive behavior is an attempt to cope with affects and to re-stabilize after narcissistic injury. The military and the police force were desperate attempts on Frank's part to balance his impulsivity by finding a containing structure, an unconscious means with which to both externalize his "badness" and seek out a force capable of controlling the part of him that internalized his father. However, these structures were insufficient and, without them, his life began to spiral out of control. Eventually he ended up in prison, the biggest container of them all.

Additionally, Frank is experiencing middle age, a narcissistic insult in its own right, which may have helped precipitate this crisis.

4. What potential pitfalls would you envision in this therapy? What would the difficulties be and what would you envision to be the source(s) of the difficulties?

In my opinion, the main pitfall in this therapy would be to miss the diagnostic complexity of this case. Antisocial personality disorder only addresses part of Frank's character pathology. The current DSM does not distinguish between antisocial personality and psychopathy. Frank also meets the criteria for narcissistic personality disorder. Ignoring the character pathology represented by both sadism and narcissism could be quite detrimental to the therapy (as well as potentially to the therapist). Additionally, I would suspect that Frank meets the criteria for "post traumatic stress disorder (PTSD)." He is also quite depressed. It is important to determine if symptoms of depression stem from a mood disorder or from characterological deficits. Case formulation and treatment would be different in each situation.

The hallmarks of antisocial personality disorder are chronic criminal behavior and disregard for the feelings of others. Frank also has a history of hurting people physically and emotionally while sometimes enjoying their suffering (sadism). Psychopaths are able to establish and maintain relationships based only on humiliation and distress. They defend themselves from unbearable affects of shame and emotional neediness by projecting what they experience as weakness onto others and then punishing them for this weakness. The punishment causes the psychopath relief, a sense of control, and emotional and sexual enjoyment which is often addictive in nature (Meloy, 1988).

Frank has significant psychopathic traits. Childhood indicators of psychopathy are the combination of bedwetting, cruelty to animals, and fire setting. Frank exhibited at least one of these. If psychopathic traits predominate, a therapy based on empathic connection will not work. However, enough contrasting indicators are present in his history that would argue for trying this form of treatment, the most important being his relationship with his wife and his honorable discharge from the military. Neither of these accomplishments is normally within the capacity of a true psychopath. Frank's intensity in relationships, his sexual behavior (including the assaults), and his sexual identity diffusion all indicate traits of borderline personality as opposed to sadism or psychopathy. There is a quality of desperation present in the description of his behaviors. The alcoholism is another indicator of instability of mood (as opposed to the more organized pathology of sadism). The level of psychopathy can be fully assessed during the second phase of treatment (see question 9).

According to the trauma literature (see Allen, 2001), women with PTSD often present with symptoms that mimic borderline personality. My experience suggests that men with PTSD present with symptoms that mimic antisocial personality. Additionally, the criteria listed in the DSM for depression often do not best describe male depression. Men tend not to get weepy; they get angry. They don't self mutilate; they become "two-fisted drinkers," act out violently, or crash their cars . If the Axis I diagnoses are not accurately assessed and represented, treatment will suffer. The true pitfall here is that Frank's presentation is so off-putting that it might deflect the therapist from seeing his underlying issues (which of course is its purpose).

5. To what level of coping, adaptation, or function would you see this patient reaching as an immediate result of therapy? What result would be long-term subsequent to the ending of therapy? (Prognosis for adaptive change?)

During the first phase of therapy (typically 12–16 weeks) I would expect to see a decrease in symptoms. Frank would appear less tense, less provocative, and less overtly hostile. He would exhibit some improved coping mechanisms such as less frequent and less severe acting-out His functioning would improve as the therapy would be focusing on his day-to-day life. However, Frank would still be lying often. The lying would serve to maintain distance from the therapist and to reduce shame. And none of this progress would be internalized. Frank would be contained primarily by his parole and the mandate to attend therapy.

The most dramatic changes occur in the client during the middle phase of psychodynamic therapy. Here, Frank would initially feel some relief that he would be able to share personal issues with someone who wants to hear them. However, as he began to talk about the major issues in his life, affect would overload Frank's defenses and he would regress. The first part of the middle phase of therapy is a frantic balancing act of attempting to hear and contain affect while simultaneously building new coping mechanisms. This is a trying period of time for both client and therapist. However, once the containers are in place, Frank's ability to verbalize will improve significantly and, for the first time, he will feel understood by someone else. The therapeutic relationship deepens dramatically during this working period, issues of transference and countertransference can be verbalized and processed, and many of Frank's pathological defenses will melt away. Trauma work begins in earnest here.

The prognosis for change depends upon how long Frank is willing to remain in therapy. If he does only some of the middle phase work, he would remain constricted affectively. There would always be pockets of the traumatization which would be triggered by various events over the course of life, as the gaps in the work break open. However, it would be quite possible that he could be generally sober, not acting out violently, having some ability to empathize with others and to control most of his urges to break the law. Still, he might commit minor crime to make money and buttress self-esteem.

If Frank stayed the course and fully worked through the impairments and deficits in his personality structure, it would be possible that he would no longer meet the criteria for antisocial or narcissistic personality disorder. Frank would have, I imagine, many interests and talents that would emerge during the second phase of therapy, activities would involve creation and not destruction; however Frank would always enjoy wheeling and dealing. I could see him becoming a leader in 12 Step programs. He would appreciate the structure and guidelines for relating with others. Frank would always have a tendency toward depression and impulsive behavior. He would always know how to swindle whomever he was dealing with. However, he would be capable of monitoring these thoughts as indicators of emotional upheaval and get help when needed.

6. What would be your timeline (duration) for therapy? What would be the frequency and duration of the sessions?

Psychodynamically based psychotherapy tends to be long-term in nature as is trauma-based treatment, defined as between 5 to 10 years. However, it is unclear from the case presentation whether Frank would be willing or even able to engage in the rigors of such a therapy. He might stay in treatment only for as long as he is mandated. In this type of work, it is always the client who determines the timeline for therapy and not the therapist.

The critical juncture in long-term therapy occurs as the beginning phase of treatment is approaching its conclusion. The focus of this phase is on establishing and strengthening the therapeutic relationship, improvement of coping skills, affect tolerance, and problem solving, all relating to day-to-day life in the present It typically takes 3 to 4 months of weekly sessions for a client to feel at ease with the therapist and to begin to experience a reduction in symptoms. These changes demonstrate that the transition to the second phase of therapy can begin. However, the severity of Frank's illness would most likely dictate a much longer beginning phase, perhaps lasting several years.

Once the transition has begun, Frank, whose primary coping strategy has been to avoid affect, faces a dilemma. If therapy stops here, he can enjoy some benefit but without the anxiety of exploring the emerging patterns of behavior and other telltale indicators that there is more to the problem than what can be addressed through a focus on symptoms alone. If Frank were no longer mandated and his wife were not complaining as loudly, he might very well stop at this point. However, many clients, after beginning to experience the relief the first few months of therapy can bring, find themselves curious about what brought them to this place in their lives. They have worked hard to accomplish these improvements and want to continue. They are confident in the therapeutic nature of the work and express a need to find peace and contentment, mind states which are predicated on a deeper understanding and acceptance of feelings and experiences. In other words, as the beginning phase of therapy ends, clients can just start to glimpse how good things might become. In this case, if they can commit emotionally, financially, and time-wise, clients will continue on. If Frank felt this way, he would commit to the therapy regardless of the mandate. The middle phase of long-term therapy typically takes years and, during exploration of particularly painful affects and experiences, it is best to meet at least twice weekly. As termination approaches, meetings can be scheduled more flexibly, sometimes less than once weekly, based on the nature of the therapeutic work (see question 14).

7. Are there specific or special techniques that you would implement in the therapy? What would they be?

The special techniques necessary for work with any client presenting with severe character pathology such as Frank's are mainly specific to the beginning phase of therapy when Frank would be at his most abrasive. The techniques' purposes are to intervene in the cycle of narcissistic injury: to protect the therapist from acting on his or her anger and to reduce Frank's reliance on enraging and distancing people.

The five main types of narcissistic assault therapists experience when working with clients with antisocial/narcissistic personality disorder are: arrogant and contemptuous behavior designed to make the therapist feel inadequate and stupid, chronic lying, constant attempts to get the therapist to violate boundaries (demandingness, entitlement, and grandiosity), the client's extreme self-absorption, and the potential for serious acting-out behavior. This fifth issue will be addressed in question 8. The most common countertransference reactions are moral indignation; anger; feeling stupid, clumsy, and unprepared; fear about the potential for danger; and a desire to be punitive, including engaging in negative judgments of the client and name-calling.

Morrison (1989) describes early experiences of traumatizing humiliation by significant others as causing a yearning in the narcissistically injured adult for absolute uniqueness and sole importance to someone else. He states that this need can be expressed either directly as assertions of entitlement, defensively as haughty aloofness and grandiosity, or affectively through rageful responses. Grandiose demands indicate the need to be unique to someone, so special that the rules don't count. Morrison views contempt as projected shame. It is important to keep in mind that Frank's attempts to distance cloak a desperate need for connection.

Special techniques with this client are methods designed to provide a balance, to address both the distancing and beckoning components of the communications. In order to remain connected to Frank and to begin to introduce him to non-narcissistic means of relating, the therapist needs to model the type of behavior he or she would want to see in Frank. These communications would include being respectful and honest with him and making comments based on his point of view. It is often effective in reducing provocative behaviors to employ a behavioral technique of praising or otherwise reinforcing positive behavior and ignoring bad behavior (unless it is serious). Limits are set in a neutral tone. Confrontation is to be avoided if at all possible until well into the middle phase of treatment when the client is able to hear it. Otherwise, all discussion will deteriorate into power struggles. On the other hand, a warm or nurturing approach at this point in the therapy is to be avoided as Frank would find it overwhelming.

During the middle phase of therapy, after a working relationship has been established, these defensive maneuvers will diminish. Any spike in provocative communications indicates that Frank has become overwhelmed by affect. It signals a breach in the therapeutic container which would best be addressed by a temporary return to the techniques of the first phase.

8. Are there special cautions to be observed in working with this patient (e.g. danger to self or others, transference, countertransference)? Are there particular resistances you would expect and how would you deal with them?

Transference, countertransference, and resistance are the lifeblood of psychodynamic therapy. It is impossible to discuss them as a separate issue. Here, I will limit my remarks about special cautions to the issue of danger, and the types of transference, countertransference, and resistance that typically appear when danger is brought into the therapeutic relationship.

It is clear from Frank's assessment that he is a dangerous man and has engaged in much abusive behavior. As a child, he also engaged in self-destructive behaviors. Frank has been retaliatory and vengeful in his interpersonal relationships. In addition, he is a substance abuser, which further increases his impulsivity and reduces his ability to make judgments. Frank knows that others perceive him as dangerous. He would probably say that he is proud of that because he would equate people fearing him with manhood, personal power, and the ability to command respect. What are the feelings (transference) that would cause Frank to need to appear so dangerous? Frank needs to feel dangerous to others because he feels so endangered himself by others. Early parental loss and severe physical and emotional abuse cause destruction of a child's interpersonal boundaries. Frank experiences the therapist as dangerous and overcompensates to ensure that no one gets close again to cause him to re-experience his childhood feelings of abject helplessness, terror, humiliation, rejection, abandonment, and pain.

Therapists listening to Frank's history would respond (countertransference) with fear, and rightfully so. Sometimes when therapists have difficulty admitting they are afraid (resistance), they will respond by provoking the client (countertransference acting-out) or they will find a way to avoid treating the client. Informing the client that one is not qualified to help him and aiding in a referral is quite appropriate. However, labeling the client as untreatable or other negative and non-clinical designations is the therapist's acting out countertransference feelings.

What is Frank resisting by engaging in dangerous behavior? Acting-out is the main coping mechanism for people with both antisocial personality disorder and substance abuse histories. Shengold (1989) states that the overstimulation an abused child experiences can only be discharged by explosive acting-out. Relational theory states that it re-creates the conditions of the original trauma within an interpersonal context (the repetition compulsion). What Frank would say by the middle phase of therapy when he was able to articulate some of his affects is that the acting-out preserved his sanity.

Prior to Frank's developing internalized means with which to contain his behavior and impulses, careful observation and management of Frank's emotional states is critical. Too much shame, fear, or anxiety may cause Frank to act out. If Frank feels safe and cared-about by his therapist, the relationship provides a counterweight to his overwhelming affects and an environment in which they can be safely communicated and processed. If the container of the therapeutic relationship is inadequate, particularly at the beginning of treatment, Frank may need a more concrete, external container for his dangerous impulses such as incarceration.

9. Are there any areas that you would choose to avoid or not address with this patient? Why?

The question of avoidance of therapeutic issues is determined by both a full clinical assessment of Frank's psychopathy and the phase of the therapy. During the beginning, focus is solely on day-to-day functioning, shoring up ego functions (decision making, judgments, affect tolerance, reduction of acting out behavior), and most importantly, establishing a therapeutic alliance. Any long-term issues are avoided here.

If Frank continued therapy beyond the first phase, then the exploratory and restorative work of the second phase can begin. Here issues of the loss of his mother; the abuse perpetuated by his family; his abuse of others and the role that violence plays for him; issues of sexual molestation and sexual identity; addictions; emotional intimacy; development and maintenance of healthy interpersonal boundaries; development of a healthy superego (a working sense of guilt); reducing criminal behavior; affects of loss, shame, humiliation, etc. can be examined and processed.

During this phase of the work, a full assessment of Frank's level of psychopathy can be ascertained. Determination of Frank's capacity in this area is made by assessment of transference and countertransference responses. If Frank were primarily narcissistic and not psychopathic, by the middle of the second phase of therapy he would no longer be trying to enrage or humiliate the therapist. He would show some genuine distress if he upset him or her. He would talk about his feelings for the therapist and how terrifying this process of attachment is. The therapist would feel as if a truce had (finally) been established and would feel far less anger and defensiveness. It would be possible to sense other affects in Frank besides rage, such as sadness, fear, and confusion. Frank would crave more closeness with his therapist. He would take steps in that direction, become scared, and quickly re-establish distance. His facial expressions would become more open and full. His tones of voice would have more nuance. His range of affect would increase and he would appear more relaxed.

However, the combination of psychopathic and narcissistic traits make Frank a quick study and he will learn what is expected of him during the first phase of therapy. He would present a facade of involvement, like his initially charming presentation. This is either movement toward a genuine engagement or an indication of the limit of his capacity. Someone with predominantly psychopathic traits is not able to forge this type of connection and, when he senses his failure, he will become enraged and attempt to humiliate and anger the therapist. (In my 7 years of working in a mental health unit of a maximum security prison, this occurred twice. However, death row inmates were not permitted therapy. I expect that if I had been permitted to see them, the incidence of true psychopathy would have occurred more frequently in my caseload.)

If Frank's psychopathic traits predominated, then second phase exploration would stop, a return to first phase work would be necessary, and therapeutic focus would remain there for the course of treatment.

10. Is medication warranted for this patient? What effect would you hope/expect the medication to have?

It would be helpful for Frank's treatment if medication were successful in reducing some of his symptoms. Unfortunately, conventional wisdom indicates that medication tends to be ineffective in treating symptoms which result from a personality disorder. There has been success in using antidepressant medications (the SSRIs) in treating symptoms of PTSD as well as for clients with substance abuse histories. A caveat in prescribing psychotropic medication to a substance abuser is the risk to the liver if the client does not remain sober and the danger of overuse or misuse of the medication. Additionally, use of medication in the treatment of character-disordered clients can reinforce their notion of externalization of control rather than a focus on their own efforts.

As mentioned in question 4, it is important to assess the nature of Frank's depression. If it stems from his character pathology, medication will not likely have much effect. However, if he is also experiencing a mood disorder (I would want to rule out bipolar disorder, major depression, and dysthymia), medication might do wonders in reducing Frank's acting-out as well as his lethality. (There is some success in prescribing medications traditionally used for bipolar disorder with clients with borderline personality, perhaps because both diagnoses are actually present.)

I would imagine that Frank would begin to experience an increase in depression during the middle phase of therapy as he begins to experience more affect. He most likely would also experience anxiety-based symptoms should he begin to explore his childhood abuse. However, most medications prescribed solely for anxiety are contraindicated for a client with a history of substance abuse. There is one which is not addictive, and some of the SSRI antidepressants are also approved to treat anxiety. It would be important to find a psychiatrist with the patience to tolerate Frank's symptoms, manner, and behavior; the expertise to address the various diagnostic questions; and the willingness to experiment with combinations of medications not traditionally tried with a client whose diagnoses are alcohol abuse and antisocial personality disorder.

Introducing medication to the treatment would likely be difficult. Frank would most likely experience the therapist's assessment as a narcissistic assault, would regress in response, and become distancing and provocative. He would most likely say things such as he is not ill, he doesn't need therapy, he is a man and can do it on his own, doesn't need a crutch, etc. He also may take the opportunity to attempt to distance himself from the psychiatrist and obtain addictive drugs. If he were to refuse to be evaluated for medication, especially during the beginning of therapy, I would avoid a power struggle over it with him. I would continue to mention its potential usefulness when appropriate and ultimately, as with all clients who are not at acute risk, Frank would be the one to make the decision.

11. What are the strengths of the patient that can be used in the therapy?

With a client such as Frank, what at first glance may appear to be a strength may be a double-edged sword and, conversely, what typically is perceived as weakness may likewise turn out to be a strength. Frank is very bright. Normally, a client's intelligence and ability to verbalize are considered assets in therapy. Frank, however, has used his intelligence to manipulate and distance people. During the assessment, for example, he used his cleverness to stymie the interviewer. This is not an asset in therapy. On the other hand, substance abuse is typically considered to be a weakness. Clients who use substances are generally considered poor candidates for therapy, so much so that many therapists will not treat a client who is actively using. Many psychopaths avoid substance use because it impairs their abilities to engage in sadistic activities. Frank's use of substances might indicate that his feelings are not completely repressed by the use of sadistic behavior as a coping mechanism. In this case, I would consider the alcoholism to be an indicator of treatability.

Another area that would typically be perceived as a weakness is Frank's motivation level. He was only minimally cooperative with the interviewer and he made it clear what he thought of the whole process. His lifestyle would indicate that he has little motivation to change. However, men do not often request therapy without an external push. In Frank's case, it would be humiliating for him to admit an internal source of motivation. He can maintain his self-image when he says he is forced to attend. Nevertheless, he could have refused to cooperate with his parole officer and instead opt to return to prison. Or, he could have left his wife rather than accede to her demands. For a client with antisocial personality disorder, I would rate Frank as showing considerable motivation during that assessment process by signing releases, participating in the assessment interview, and particularly by completing the psychological testing.

Another perceived area of weakness is Frank's history of relationships, including his marriage. He married a woman much younger than he, told her little about himself, and when he became enraged, destroyed a valued possession of hers. However, his marriage also can be seen as a strength. Frank has been able to maintain a relationship with his wife such that she never reported feeling physically unsafe. She felt comfortable pressuring him both to go to therapy and to permit the interviewer to obtain background information. Given his history, this is remarkable. It indicates enormous control on his part, trust in her, as well as a significant commitment to maintaining his marriage. It demonstrates that he is capable of engaging in a relationship which is a source of support and nurturing without his having to completely destroy it or her. And most importantly, Frank is a survivor. He survived a horrific childhood with his sanity intact and without killing anyone. Tenacity is a strength in this type of therapy.

12. How would you address limits, boundaries, and limit-setting with this patient?

As transference and countertransference are the lifeblood of psychodynamic therapy, so are limits and boundaries its skin. They are the containers that hold everything in place. Properly set limits provide the same communication function with severely character-disordered clients as interpretation does with neurotic clients. They facilitate bringing the unconscious to consciousness, from id to ego. Id impulses are dangerous as they are out of conscious control and unable to be articulated. In this sense, the client's need for limits is also his search for safety.

Boundaries separate one individual from another and the therapeutic relationship from other types of bonds. They also contain and protect the therapeutic relationship and its participants. Limit setting is the means with which the protection is established and maintained. Frank has never experienced healthy interpersonal boundaries. His were continually violated by his father when he was a child and his own aggressive behavior was never confronted or contained by his other caretakers. Frank continually violates others' boundaries. He has no skin. He is hemorrhaging.

But the limits which will contain him must be set with care, patience, and respect for Frank's internal world. Frank makes this endeavor extremely difficult. He is verbally provocative, physically intimidating, and hostile. He responds this way because he would feel most vulnerable in this situation. He is forced to attend therapy, face divorce, or return to prison. He signed releases so that his background and level of dysfunction are known to a stranger whose purpose it is to judge him. He is not able to maintain control in the ways which he knows. He cannot be physically aggressive, run scams, or steal and disappear. He has never been this exposed except when he was very young. It would feel that dangerous to him. Frank is unable to verbalize the desperation stemming from his sense of danger or his need for safety and connection. If the limits are set properly, they will contain his impulses and provocative behavior and transform them into affect-bearing words, a much safer and more effective coping mechanism.

An example would best describe this process. Joe, a client serving a prison sentence for manslaughter, demanded at the beginning of each of his weekly therapy sessions to use my phone to call his family. Each time I said no and gently explained that I was not permitted to do that. He became enraged. He would glare and accuse me of withholding care and trying to "make him go off." We would then continue the session. After about a year of this, one day he no longer asked. When I questioned why, he said that if I wouldn't let him use the phone, it must mean that I actually wanted to talk to him.

Frank's internalization of healthy interpersonal boundaries, this vital aspect of self; must be experienced in order for it to be learned. The only way to accomplish this is through precisely applied limits. Only then will Frank be able to internalize these changes, build boundaries for himself, and be able to locate and respect those of others.

13. Would you want to involve significant others in the treatment? Would you use out-of-session work (homework) with this patient? What homework would you use?

Significant others could be involved in the treatment if Frank felt it would be helpful. However, Frank must be the one to decide. A client with a history of severe trauma will experience the therapist's unilateral decision to add people to the therapy as a boundary violation. Frank needs to feel that the therapeutic relationship belongs to him. Generally, if Frank were to request family or couples work, it would most likely not occur during the first phase of treatment. He would need to know that he can control his therapist's access to information about him. The presence of others at this early phase of treatment would most likely increase his sense of humiliation and vulnerability.

It may be useful during the second phase of therapy for Frank to invite his wife for some couples work. Experiencing from an outsider's perspective the changes in a client during the second phase of therapy (with no clear understanding of the process) can be bewildering for family members. In addition, Frank might want the support of the therapy environment to voice concerns or feelings to his wife. If Frank requested that his wife accompany him on an ongoing basis, I would do so only as an adjunct to the individual therapy, not to usurp it, as the request might be made as a defense to shift the focus from him.

Alternately, the thought of having anyone else involved in the therapy might be quite threatening to Frank, particularly if he has just established what feels to him like a safe and nurturing relationship. He might fear that a relative would take the therapist away from him, as so many of his caregivers were taken from him in childhood. All of these factors would need to be carefully assessed in making this decision. I would verbalize them to Frank and then make the decision with him. This intervention enhances his decision-making skills as well as permits him the experience of shared control.

Research indicates that writing assignments such as journal entries can facilitate the reprocessing of traumatic memories and feelings (Allen, 2001). It also provides a cognitive container for affect. Frank is intelligent and, if he enjoys writing, homework such as this would further the treatment. However, power struggles with clients over homework are to be avoided, particularly with someone such as Frank. Homework can also represent school, which raises issues of failure, compliance, control, judgment, and humiliation, all of which reinforce childhood trauma and are central issues in sociopathic personality organization. It also assumes literacy. I would assign homework with care, and only if the client continued to do it willingly and reported that it seemed worthwhile. In addition to keeping a journal, workbooks on childhood trauma which contain exercises teaching the client to label and express affect, self soothe, and find alternate coping strategies might be a helpful adjunct to the therapy.

14. What would be the issues to be addressed in termination? How would termination and relapse prevention be structured?

Issues to be addressed in termination would depend on the type of ending that occurs. Less than optimal ends to the therapy include Frank's dropping out or his re-incarceration. In these cases, the main issue to be addressed is to ensure the potential for Frank's return. Toward this end, outreach can take place by written communication. I would describe to Frank what I saw as successes in his treatment and I would encourage him to contact me in the future. If Frank left treatment when he could only show the disdainful, humiliating, and aggressive parts of himself and continued to push limits throughout the therapy, I would write to inform him that the therapy had officially ended. I would indicate (in a compassionate and respectful tone) that there were problems in how it went, and I would say that if he were willing to address his behavior I would be willing to meet with him again if he so chose.

If Frank's therapy were successful, the termination phase would occur over a long period of time. Termination reworks the major aspects of the therapy itself. It also causes the client to revisit past losses within the context of the current loss. These issues and affects must be contained during the termination phase so as to avoid regression and acting-out. Acting-out behavior may include dropping out or behaving in such a way as to force the therapy to continue.

The final task of termination is internalization of the therapist. Frank must be able to take in as his own the functions that the therapist performed for him as well as any aspects of himself that he projected to the therapist. An example of internalization is when clients describe being able to hear their therapist in their own minds, what he or she would say in a difficult or stressful situation.

The structure of meetings during this phase would depend on Frank's needs and wishes. During the period of intense work on affects relating to loss, sessions would most likely increase in frequency, but as the end nears, clients often prefer to meet less frequently as a means to practice being without the therapist. My experience of successful termination with long-term clients is that the boundary is flexible. Clients can and often do return from time to time to work on specific issues, or they write, drop by, or sometimes refer their children to see me. Although the physical meetings may have ceased, the attachment remains quite alive, for both of us.

Relapse prevention is a cognitive therapy-based program of shoring up ego functions. These concepts would be introduced at the beginning of treatment and worked on throughout its course. By the end, Frank would have a working knowledge of relapse prevention techniques and would be applying the principles himself. Relapse prevention concepts provide a good segue to self-help programs if Frank were not already attending.

15. What do you see as the hoped for mechanisms of change for this patient, in relative importance?

In a psychodynamic model of treatment, the mechanism of change is the therapeutic relationship itself. The factors within it which produce change are the holding environment; work on ego functions; verbalization with appropriate affect, referred to as "working through;" and most importantly, empathic attunement between therapist and client. Resulting changes in the client include an increase in the capacity to tolerate affect, strengthening of ego functions, reduction in impulsivity, and improvements in interpersonal boundaries and the capacity for intimacy.

However, clients with severe character pathology by definition do not have the capacity to verbalize affect, attune empathically, or work through their issues. Therapists working with this client population must work with primitive and latent forms of communication before the client will be able to engage in the more complex mechanisms of change listed above. The most important and sometimes only mechanism of change with a deeply impaired client is the repetition compulsion. The concept, introduced by Freud (1915), happens when the repetition of behavior substitutes for conscious recollection. Russell (1998) describes the repetition compulsion as representing the scar tissue of interruptions of attachment, attachments the person needed in the service of emotional growth. It is inversely related to intimacy and occurs in lieu of grief.

The repetition compulsion is operating when one person's affects related to past trauma are experienced by a significant other within a current interpersonal relationship. Traumatic events, most likely relating to inadequate nurture or abuse, are triggered unconsciously during the course of an emotionally close relationship. The traumatized person does not have the capacity to differentiate the affect as coming from the past. It is intolerable and unconsciously dispersed through repression, acting-out, and projection to his or her partner. The partner identifies with it and reacts accordingly.

The repetition compulsion, like projective identification, is a universally experienced aspect of relating. The concept, which appears arcane and theoretical in abstract form, is instantly recognizable when applied to daily life and our intimate relationships. It is operating any time you keep having the same argument about a behavior with the same person over and over again. It feels completely out of control and seems solely the fault of the other, who appears to take a perverse pleasure in making you miserable. (Think of your spouse, your mother, your teenaged son, your boss, the boss before this one, and the one before that, or if all else fails, your ex.) Like the protagonist of a horror movie, you desperately want it to stop but no matter what you do or how hard you try to change it, despite all efforts, it proceeds as if it had a life of its own, because it does.

In the therapeutic relationship, the client who is repeating compulsively creates conditions by his behavior where the therapist experiences as his or her own what the client should have been feeling in the past (Tansey &

Burke, 1989). To the therapist, the verbal exchange feels stuck, lifeless, pressured and manipulative. He or she feels pulled to react in a certain way, as if at the wheel of a car on the highway whose tire has just blown. It suddenly feels very unsafe in the room, as if something just out of reach, unpleasant and perhaps dangerous, were rapidly unfolding. To the client, although frustratingly familiar, it also seems completely outside of his control. He is unaware of wanting what results. Repetition compulsions can be enactments of simple affects or, as the therapy progresses, they can represent extraordinarily complex and pathological dynamics. What is most confusing for both therapist and client is that until it is rendered, delivered into consciousness, it remains inscrutable, happening over and over until conditions within the therapeutic relationship are such that it can be deciphered.

Russell (n.d.) said that psychopathology can be measured by the severity and malignancy of the repetition compulsion and by the degree to which the treatment relationship is threatened. Frank would rate high on this scale. His verbal interactions and behavior demand that the therapist play the role of the protagonist as Frank imposes his own horror movie on the therapeutic relationship. How can this predicament possibly be a mechanism of change?

Firstly, while the repetition compulsion does function to repress and project intolerable affect, it also simultaneously propels it forward into the therapeutic relationship, delivering the affect to the person most capable of understanding, tolerating, and containing it. It is a communication tool which conveys its message much more powerfully than words ever could. Reliance on the repetition compulsion represents the client's hope that this interaction might end differently than before.

Secondly, it permits a comprehensive assessment of the client's functioning and major deficits, but it does so in a manner that is the reverse of the typical way in which a therapist makes an assessment. Normally, a therapist takes a history and learns of the client's difficulties from the information and the client's presentation. In Frank's case, the therapist will learn of his issues by his behaving in ways that recreate the themes of his trauma for the therapist to experience (Gorkin, 1996). Frank creates conditions in which his therapist will feel the levels of humiliation, rage, and despair that he felt as a child. Frank cannot describe these in words but countertransference will make it abundantly clear to the therapist. An additional benefit is that this mode of communication is lie-proof.

If the therapist succeeds in experiencing these affects and understanding them as belonging to the client, a response can be fashioned that is non-retaliatory and provides containment for both the behavior and the affect.

Often, because the affect is communicated behaviorally, the response from the therapist needs to be in the form of a limit. An intervention which assumes that the behavior is conscious will be ineffective. The client will experience it as a narcissistic assault which will recreate the original traumatic conditions. (An example is Frank's responses concerning his need for treatment, his alcohol use, and his employment history.)

After many, many of these interactions, the client will learn to experience the affect as contained within the therapeutic relationship and will begin to be able to tolerate it. Here, the client experiences a reparative relationship for the first time. And within this safety and security, repetition compulsions can be transformed from unconscious fragmented id impulses to conscious and fully experienced emotion. Only now, when the client is able to verbalize, will the therapist learn of the specifics of what he or she already knows. The events can then be retained and reintegrated into memory as past experience (Chu, 1991) as interpersonal boundaries are strengthened. Each time a trauma represented by a repetition compulsion is delivered into consciousness, grief must be experienced for the attachment that did not happen when it was needed. The grieving begins the process of working through, where interventions can now be based on consciously experienced affect.

Joe, the client in question 12, provides a good example of communication in the form of a repetition compulsion. It was impossible to determine the nature of the conflict from his demand for a phone call, but his affective state could be ascertained by exploring my countertransference responses. I was very guarded with Joe, feeling that he might easily misread anything I said. I dreaded the weekly request for the call and each week, without fail, he forced my hand. His accusation that I was trying to make him "go off" felt crazy to me. Why would I want to make a man who killed another lose control of his temper? It was impossible to explain this to him. I tried. He sneered. But he abided by the limit and returned each week so that we could re-engage in this interaction anew. Once the issue of the phone call was resolved, Joe was able to relate the events which led up to his crime. Joe, badly sexually abused as a child, mistook a hostile sexualized gesture made toward him by another man as a homosexual attack (he later understood it to be an attempt to humiliate him), became overwhelmed with terror and rage, and killed him. Each week in demanding the phone call of me, he projected the intolerable affects which led up to his offense: the misreading, the dreaded interaction, the forcing of my hand, his projected feeling that I was trying to make him "go off." It was only when Joe experienced that I could tolerate this explosive affect, his feeling that I really wanted to talk to him, could it be permitted into consciousness so that he could see the pattern of interactions and begin to make sense of his behavior.

REFERENCES/SUGGESTED READING

Allen, Jon G. (2001). *Traumatic relationships and serious mental disorders.* Chichester, England: John Wiley & Sons.

Balint, Michael. (1968). *The basic fault.* London: Tavistock. Reprinted 1979. New York: Brunner/Mazel.

Bowlby, John. (1982). *Attachment* (2nd ed.). New York: Basic Books.

Bromberg, Philip M. (1998). *Standing in the spaces: Essays on clinical process, trauma & dissociation.* Hillsdale, NJ: The Analytic Press.

Buckley, Peter (Ed.). (1986). *Essential papers on object relations.* New York: New York University Press.

Casement, Patrick J. (1985). *Learning from the patient.* New York: Guilford Press.

Chu, James A. (1991). The repetition compulsion revisited: Reliving dissociated trauma. *Psychotherapy, 28,* 327–332.

Coen, Stanley. (2002). *Affect tolerance in patient and analyst.* Northvale, NJ: Jason Aronson.

Crittendon, Patricia McKinsey. (1995). Attachment and psychopathology. In S. Goldberg, R. Muir, & J. Kerr (Eds.), *Attachment theory: Social, developmental, and clinical perspectives.* Hillsdale, NJ: Analytic Press.

Culow, Christopher. (2001). Attachment, narcissism and the violent couple. In Culow, C. (Ed.), *Adult attachment and couple psychotherapy: The Secure base in practice and research.* London: Brunner-Routledge.

Fairbairn, W.R.D. (l952). *Psychoanalytic studies of the personality.* London: Tavistock. Reprinted 1992. London: Routledge.

Freud, Sigmund. (1915). Remembering, repeating and working-through. *Standard Edition,* 12, 147–156.

Gorkin, Michael. (1996). *The uses of countertransference.* Norvale, NJ: Jason Aronson.

Grotstein, James. (1981). *Splitting and projective identification.* Northvale, NJ: Jason Aronson.

Hedges, Lawrence E. (2000). *Terrifying transferences: Aftershocks of childhood trauma.* Northvale, NJ: Jason Aronson.

Luntz, Barbara K., & Widom, Cathy Spatz. (1994). APD in abused and neglected children grown up. *American Journal of Psychiatry,* 151, 670–674.

Meloy, J. Reid. (1988). *The psychopathic mind: Origins, dynamics and treatment.* Northvale, NJ: Jason Aronson.

Mitchell, Stephen A. (1988). *Relational concepts in psychoanalysis: An integration.* Cambridge, MA: Harvard University Press.

Moore, B., & Fine, B. (Eds.). (1990). *Psychoanalytic terms and concepts.* New Haven, CT: American Psychoanalytic Association and Yale University Press.

Morrison, Andrew P. (1989). *Shame: The underside of narcissism.* Hillsdale, NJ: Analytic Press.

Roth, Loren H. (Ed.). (1987). *Clinical treatment of the violent person.* New York: Guilford.

Russell, Paul L. (1998). The role of paradox in the repetition compulsion. In I.G. Teicholz & D. Kreigman (Eds.), *Trauma, repetition, and affect regulation: The works of Paul Russell.* New York: The Other Press.

Russell, Paul L. (n.d.). *The theory of the crunch.* Unpublished manuscript.

Shengold, Leonard. (1989). *Soul murder: The effects of childhood abuse and deprivation.* New Haven, CT: Yale University Press.

Tansey, Michael J., & Burke, Walter F. (1989). *Understanding countertransference: From proiective identification to empathy.* Hillsdale, NJ: Analytic Press.

Van der Kolk, Bessel A. (1989). The compulsion to repeat the trauma: Re-enactment, revictimization and masochism. *Psychiatric Clinics of North America* 12, 389–411.

Wilson, John. (1989). *Trauma, transformation and healing: An integrative approach to theory. Research and post-traumatic therapy.* New York: Brunner/Mazel.

Winnicott, DW. (1972). *Holding and interpretation.* New York: Grove Press.

Wurmser, Leon. (1978). *The hidden dimension: Psychodynamics in compulsive drug use.* Northvale, NJ: Jason Aronson.

CHAPTER 4

Adlerian Psychotherapy

Michael Maniacci

I. Describe your treatment model.

Adlerian psychotherapy is based upon the work of the Viennese psychiatrist Alfred Adler, a colleague of Sigmund Freud at the turn of the twentieth century. Although he was one of the original members of Freud's "inner circle," the Vienna Psychoanalytic Society's first president, and founding coeditor of their journal, Adler soon developed a system of psychotherapy and a philosophy of human nature which was very different from Freud's (Hoffman, 1994). In order to understand how contemporary Adlerians (sometimes referred to as Individual Psychologists) understand human nature and practice psychotherapy, a brief discussion of the fundamental assumptions of Individual Psychology (IP) is needed (Adler, 1956; Mosak & Shulman, 1967).

People are viewed from a holistic perspective. The parts are not given greater attention than the whole. Clinically, that means that we do not necessarily focus upon concepts such as the ego, the unconscious, emotions, or symptoms, as these are "parts" of the individual. Rather the Individual Psychologist focuses on the broader picture of the person or "individual." While we are interested in the *causes* of behavior, we place far greater emphasis upon the *purposes* of behavior. Teleology is key to our system. We examine the goals people set for themselves, both in their immediate and long-range future.

We believe in *soft determinism,* that is, while we acknowledge that within a certain range of probabilities "A leads to B," we also know that many times "A leads to C (or D, or X, etc.)." Human nature is not static, and humans are capable of not only responding to their internal and external environments, they are capable of influencing them as well.

That leads to our next assumption, *creativity*. While the concepts of free will and choice are often considered taboo within the realm of academic and clinical psychology and psychiatry, Adlerians have long emphasized that individuals choose their responses to their environments, even if we admit (as noted above) that they sometimes are extremely limited in the range of their choices. We view individuals as co-creators of their world.

Phenomenology is our next assumption. People are more influenced by their perceptions of the situation than by the situation itself. Clinically, we are not as much interested in what happens to individuals as we are in what they believe happens to them and the meaning they ascribe to it.

We view people within a *social context*. All problems have the potential of becoming social problems, and while we may focus upon an individual's belief system, we will go to great lengths to demonstrate to that person the interpersonal effects and consequences of maintaining that particular set of beliefs.

Adlerian psychology is a *field theory*. We are not as much interested in categorizing symptoms as we are in understanding their context. People may be depressed, but knowing where they are depressed, with whom, for how long, what makes the depression worse or better, and so forth, is much more fascinating to us than simply knowing that the individual is depressed.

We stress a *psychology of use*. While what we have is important, Adlerians are more interested in the use we make of what we have, particularly what social use people make of their symptoms.

Adlerian therapy is primarily *idiographic and multimodal*. That is, we place considerable value upon the individual case and its particular manifestation. While we do explore nomothetic principles, we much rather understand not the general rules of the case but how this particular case manifests the general principles we see as underlying our system. As part of the idiographic assumption, we need to tailor our treatment approach to the particulars of the individual case. In any one day—and sometimes with any one client—Adlerians may use behavioral approaches, approaches that are somewhat psychoanalytic, then switch to a behavioral focus, and maybe then to a cognitive focus (Maniacci, 1999).

Finally, we see *motivation* as a striving from a perceived minus situation to a perceived plus. People grow and are always striving towards subjectively interpreted goals. When confronted with a challenge to their striving, individuals will select various means to overcome perceived areas of deficit.

Adlerians have pioneered and currently make extensive use of individual, group, and couple and family therapy formats, and have long been advocates of brief therapy (Hoffman, 1994). We see psychotherapy as a collaborative enterprise in which therapist and client are equals. Pragmatically, that means that while clinicians may be experts in psychology and psychotherapy, clients are experts when it comes to themselves and their lives. Both must bring their knowledge to the consulting room, and both must work together to reach their mutually established goals.

Psychotherapy for us entails teaching patients to be more at ease with themselves and their social world. They should move through life with a more pro-social orientation and a greater sense of confidence and clarity. Ideally, they should leave therapy more prepared to constructively contribute to their world than to non-constructively or destructively demand that their world give to them.

II. What clinical skills are necessary to work with this patient?

The clinical skills or attributes most essential to Adlerian psychotherapy are varied and complex. Flexibility, a general sense of usefulness to humanity, empathy, and courage are just some of the keys to our approach. An exploration into each will hopefully clarify their meaning.

Individual Psychologists must be flexible. We work with a wide range of people in varied formats and with a multitude of issues. While we are very consistent in our adherence to the basic assumptions, the techniques we utilize in our psychotherapy vary according the needs of the situation. The technique must not violate the assumptions, and as long as it does not, we will use it. As noted above, with a few (admittedly controversial) exceptions, it is NOT the technique itself which is of issue, but the use clinicians make of it that counts. There IS a sense of usefulness to humanity that Adlerians characterize as community feeling, or social interest (Adler, 1956). We generally believe that the social imbeddedness of people is innate, that we are social creatures, and that the better adjusted we are to that fact, the better off we are. The needs of the group should be intertwined with our own, to such an extent that (ideally) they are inseparable. In short, what is good for me should be good for everyone, and vice versa.

Adlerian psychology can come across as somewhat moralistic, and counterbalancing the psychotherapist's emphasis upon fostering community feeling is the strong emphasis Adlerians place upon empathy. To paraphrase Alfred Adler (1956), therapists are encouraged to see with the eyes of another, hear with the ears of another, and feel with the heart of another. While we strongly and emphatically ask clients to be responsible for what they do, we also stress understanding how they feel, what they think, and why they feel and think the way that they do. Compassion is important, and a good therapeutic relationship may be one of the first steps in fostering social interest.

We see discouragement as the cardinal feature of all psychological dysfunction. People become discouraged in their ability to move towards their goals in pro-social ways. We therefore want to encourage clients to re-engage in a cooperative way. Adlerian psychotherapists need to demonstrate courage, or as one Adlerian defines it, the willingness to risk even if the outcome is uncertain (Mosak, 1995). By demonstrating hope, love, faith, and the courage to be imperfect, clinicians can model good interpersonal relations for their clients (Mosak).

Frank J. is a challenging client. Adler (1930/1976) was very interested in the issue of criminality and criminals, and Rudolf Dreikurs (1977) described the criminal personality, or what would now be called the antisocial personality disorder (ASP), in some detail. In his view, ASPs, as well as all personality-disordered individuals, lack common sense, that is, the ability to think in a consensual, cooperative manner. They are not psychotic, but rather they follow their own private sense, or logic, to such an extent that they typically violate the rules of society. They grow up in an environment in which they believe that their private logic is common sense. They believe that how they think is how others think, and when they discover that others do not think their way, ASPs are frequently initially amazed and then contemptuous of how "naive" others are. Their life styles, or personalities, form these fundamental beliefs (Sperry & Mosak, 1996). Typical themes might include:

It is a dog eat dog world.
I should be top dog, without limits, and totally free to do what I want to do.
Other people can't be trusted. They want to fence me in and limit my freedom.

Their methods of operation vary, depending upon the type of situation they grew up in, their physical make-up, and current context. In general, Dreikurs (1977) detailed three types of ASPs: (a) The Ruling Types. These individuals became tyrants, "hit men," or dictators. Their preferred methods of operation are to attempt overt control through domination, intimidation, and force. They attain their freedom through violence. (b) The Self-Indulgent Types. These individuals become addicts, confidence artists, and master manipulators. Their preferred methods of operation are to develop excellent social skills, quick minds, and smooth communication skills in order to get their way. They attain their freedom through using people or substances or both. (c) The Organically Impaired Types. These individuals typically manifest mostly Ruling Types of behavior, but for special reasons. Because of structural central nervous system dysfunction, such as mental retardation and inadequate early training, or not being given the necessary early environmental support and attention, these people frequently broke society's rules because they did not understand them. Because their early environments either ignored their organic impairment or were ignorant or indifferent to it, these individuals started out with "two strikes against them," so to speak. The troubles they get into are a combination of an inability to control themselves and a lack of a supportive atmosphere which could have taught them or sheltered them from the adverse affects their impairments had upon them (Adler, 1930/1976).

Frank seems to have elements of all three types. Given the abusive background he had, and the history of violence his father demonstrated, it would not be surprising to find structural neuropsychological or neurological damage with neuropsychological testing. This damage might be secondary to early physical abuse, perhaps even a hereditary factor. Since the evidence for such an hypothesis is scarce at best, I will approach the case emphasizing that he is a combination of the Ruling and Self-Indulgent Types. Primarily, in my clinical judgment, he is mostly the Ruling Type.

1. What would be your therapeutic goal? What is the primary goal? The secondary goal?

The primary goal of all Adlerian psychotherapy is to foster a sense of community feeling. Idiographically, I would want to try to teach Frank to be more considerate of others and to be far less violent. Specifically, I would offer the following:

- "Victim" identification. I would attempt to have Frank put himself in the place of those he has victimized and would victimize. I would want to see how empathic he is and eventually could become.
- I would attempt to increase his optimism. This is not an idealistic attempt on my part, though admittedly it is a challenging one. His impulsivity is (in part) most likely related to a profound discouragement and pessimism about his future. Because of his doubts about his future, he may believe that he had "better get it now." The more optimistic Frank may become about his future, perhaps he will be less likely to live solely for today.

- Teach him to examine the consequences of his actions. Frank has not learned from his actions, nor does he see the relationship between what he does and what is done to him.
- Bring his substance-abuse issues into focus and establish a contract for either decreasing or stopping his drinking, including possible referral to a substance-abuse program, consultation with a substance-abuse specialist, or the use of a Rational Recovery or Alcoholics Anonymous group (see point number 12, below).

Other, more specific goals will be addressed throughout subsequent parts of this project.

2. What further information would you want to have to assist in structuring this patient's treatment? Are their specific assessment tools you would use? What would be the rationale for using these tools?

While we have much of the data we would need to conduct a life-style assessment of Frank, I would like to have some additional information. For instance, I would need to have some early recollections (Shulman & Mosak, 1988). These are single, specific recollections he would recall from before the age of 10 years. A recent ASP of mine gave as one of his early recollections the following incident:

Age 7 years. We were eating Thanksgiving dinner, gathered around the table. It was snowing outside, and our neighbor took out his snow-blower and began clearing his driveway. We heard something like a scream, ran to the window, and saw that he had tried to clear something from the machine and gotten his hand caught in it. Most vivid moment: The blood shooting out onto the white snow. Feeling: It was cool, exciting.

Interpreted projectively, this client does not feel compassion nor empathy for his neighbors. Life is an exciting place where harm coming to others leads to satisfaction for him. In a cold world, other people's·pain brings excitement to him.

While no one early recollection is enough, 8–10 can show clear patterns and trends inherent in a client's belief system. Frank's early recollections would prove invaluable.

Since I am a clinical psychologist, in addition to a life-style assessment, I would probably want some psychological testing. Intelligence testing and neuropsychological screening, objective personality testing and projective testing, especially with the Rorschach Inkblot Test, would prove quite beneficial. (Since I would reinterpret the data from the previous testing with the

Rorschach and MMPI along Adlerian lines, I might simply reexamine the raw data from the original testing.)

A hypothetical summary of his psychosocial history, what Adlerians refer to as a Summary of Family Constellation (Powers & Griffith, 1987; Shulman & Mosak, 1988), might sound like this:

Frank is the elder of two boys and psychologically a first-born who grew up in an abusive, oppressive atmosphere where the dominant family values were power, control, and getting your way no matter what the cost. Father was a tyrant who ruled the house without mercy, and he could be abusive and humiliating when it came to discipline. Frank never knew a lot about his mother, and had a series of women in his early life that were both transitory and ineffectual. Frank began to believe that life was unfair, power was important, and people's feelings were insignificant. He all too often saw the pain his brother experienced and decided that feelings were a hindrance, and therefore he trained himself to avoid them. He did the only thing he felt he could do in order to survive: He joined forces with the enemy. If he couldn't beat his father, he could imitate him, and that he did with cold precision. Life for Frank became a matter of overcoming challenges and proving that he could survive whatever was thrown at him, and when his father failed to offer him enough challenges, Frank went out and sought them, constantly attempting to test his will, his nerves, against life and its dangers, and thereby prove that what didn't kill him made him stronger. Like Father, he believed that he was a real man because he was rough, tough, and unwilling to take anything from anyone.

I would present this summary to Frank, ask him to edit it, revise it, and join me in its elaboration, and (by and large) share the formal testing results with him. We would work together on the life-style assessment, and try to figure out why he came to the conclusions he came to.

3. What is your conceptualization of this patient's personality, behavior, affective state, and cognitions?

While the life-style assessment would provide the basis for an assessment of Frank's personality, behavior, affective state, and cognitions, a more detailed analysis could be presented. First of all, since one of our basic assumptions is holism, divisions such as those articulated in this section would not be very meaningful for an Adlerian. Frank's personality is inseparable from his behavior, affective state, and cognitions. We would treat them as a whole. As (almost) an academic exercise, we could break down the above assessment this way:

- Long-range personality goals: To be free, dominant, and in control.
- Frequent short-range (immediate) goals: To intimidate. Power and revenge would be the frequent immediate goals for which he would strive. Intimacy and commitment would be avoided, since they might tie him down and make him vulnerable, for if he commits, he could get hurt.
- Frequent emotions: While in any specific instance, he might experience any emotion, primarily he would probably focus upon pleasure, pain-avoidance, and apathy (if he doesn't actively care about anything, no one can control him; the purpose of apathy is to remain beyond anyone's control).

His cognitions could best be described after seeing and interpreting his early recollections. However, in general, they probably would be very similar to the beliefs Dreikurs (1977) identified as part of the ASP's belief system.

4. What potential pitfalls would you envision in this therapy? What would the difficulties be and what would you envision being the sources of these difficulties?

The potential pitfalls in this therapy are numerous. For instance, Frank does not trust, and psychotherapy involves trust. I would have to be very careful not to speak his language too mechanically, for he would probably see me as trying to control him or limit his freedom. Similarly, we would have to be very clear about confidentiality, informed consent, duty to warn, and other such guidelines. This case could be a management nightmare, for so many people could be involved. Keeping the lines of communication clear would be challenging.

Frank sees life as one filled with pain when you are not "top dog." He probably would have a hard time letting me take over, yet to let him be in charge might prove frustrating.

Honesty and frankness are not frequent bedfellows with these clients. In working with ASPs, it is easy to confuse collaboration with manipulation, both from clients and clinicians. I find I always want to be "clever" with these individuals, and sometimes I just end up being foolish. It is difficult to beat them at their own game, and to try to do so usually ends up in a mess.

Finally, the social implications of Frank's behavior are far-reaching and potentially dangerous. Such work frequently places therapists in precarious positions, such as having to decide if the particular course of a discussion might end up with ASPs getting mad, storming out of sessions, and taking out their anger against others, even against the therapists themselves. Adlerians, as much as anybody, are fully aware of the social implications of symptomatic behavior.

5. To what level of coping would you see this patient reaching as an immediate result of therapy? What result would be long-term subsequent to the ending of therapy?

Adlerians tend to not do prognosis. In most instances, clinical prognosis leads to a sort of self-fulfilling prophecy in that clinicians look to find what they expect to be there. Such a use of prognosis I find very unhelpful.

When prognosis is used in order anticipate potential pitfalls and traps that need to be avoided, and in order to plan for constructive remediation strategies when they arise, then it IS very helpful. For instance, some psychotherapists will say that Frank has a poor prognosis. To state it that way is to establish a mind set that anticipates failure. Most Adlerians would prefer to say that Frank will be challenging. The issues identified in point number 4 above (potential pitfalls) could be anticipated and discussed with Frank. His cooperation could be elicited in order to brainstorm about how to handle such challenges if and when they arrive.

6. What would be your timeline? What would be the frequency and duration of the sessions?

I would prefer weekly individual sessions for the initial phase of therapy. After some time has elapsed and some stability has been attained, I would probably put him in weekly group psychotherapy, with individual sessions reducing to every other week. Couples and family therapy would be used as needed (see point number 13, below). A literature review shows that psychotherapy with personality disordered individuals frequently takes some time, and I could foresee 2 years of such work (e.g., Beck, Freeman, & Associates, 1990; Benjamin, 1996).

Since stage one of Adlerian psychotherapy involves building and maintaining a relationship, Frank's input would be required in all of the debate about frequency and duration. A complication is that neither Frank nor I are complete masters of our fates: There could be legal implications and various law enforcement personnel may want their input. This could be used to our mutual advantage, however, by giving us a "mutual enemy" to work against (see point number 12, below).

7. Are there specific techniques you would implement in the therapy? What would they be?

I could write a volume on this, and many clinicians have already done so. There are many techniques I would want to use (Mosak & Maniacci, 1998). Specifically, the techniques would revolve around two primary poles: confrontation/reeducation and support.

Frank is withholding. Given his history, this is understandable. Without some confrontation, this treatment would most likely evolve into a mutual admiration society with Frank spewing forth platitudes and flattering the therapist, and the therapist regurgitating some such similar canned phrases. Frank is a dangerous man; he has hurt numerous people, including those that have tried to help him, and every year he seems to become more and more adept at plying his pathology. The group format would prove invaluable in pressing him to examine his private logic. I would need a group with strong members, some of whom are much farther along in their treatment than Frank. The more they call him on his game playing, the greater the opportunity to teach him something. The more they confront and prepare him to learn, the more I could be supportive, encouraging, and empathic: "Yeah, I know Frank is a shark, but can you blame him? Look at what he had to do to survive."

This dialectic of confront/teach and support would be hard for any one therapist to do in individual psychotherapy. Fortunately, Adlerians have been advocates of multiple psychotherapy, the use of two therapists with one client (Dreikurs, Shulman, & Mosak, 1984). In this case, I would find it essential. One therapist, typically and ideally an older, senior colleague, could confront and teach, while the younger, more peer-like therapist could support and empathize.

In addition, Frank would strike me as someone with whom imagery would play a key role. With many ASPs, behavioral rehearsal of new skills is required, and the use of imagery and role playing would facilitate the process. One type of imagery technique would be restructuring his early recollections (Kopp, 1995; Maniacci, 1996). I would ask him to recall one of his distressing memories, either in individual sessions or group, and we would reenact it. I would then attempt to have him restructure the memory until it came out the way he wanted it. As is typical with many personality-disordered individuals, the process is quite difficult, for they keep recreating the same basic theme with only slight variation (Maniacci). With prompting and patience, Frank would eventually change his memory to a more pro-social, constructive version. A link could then be made to a current situation in which he is responding in much the same manner, and his new skills acquired from his childhood reconstruction could be then applied to the current problem.

Another technique I have used involves audio or video taping sessions and reviewing them with clients. In either individual or group sessions, this can facilitate learning and begin to allow Frank to "step outside" his style and view it from another's perspective.

8. Are there special cautions to be observed in working with this patient? Are there any particular resistances you would expect, and how would you deal with them?

As noted previously, there are many cautions I would take with this case. There is an obvious duty to warn issue which must be kept foremost in the clinician's mind. Confidentiality would need to be discussed and clarified in advance with Frank, for he needs to know what the implications are of his telling me certain "facts" or intentions. I would seek out and utilize a senior colleague for supervision and a "reality check," for this case could get quite complicated. And once again, my role with outside agencies, such as law enforcement officials, would need to be spelled out well in advance and agreed to by all, especially Frank.

With regard to transference issues, Adlerians do not see the need to develop transference neuroses with patients (besides, with clients like Frank, such issues are typically moot, even from a traditional psychoanalytic perspective). We conceptualize transference as the consistency of the life-style. In short, we believe that Frank's belief system will be evident both in therapy and out of therapy. Why should we expect him to behave any differently in treatment with me than outside of treatment with anyone else? I would have to watch for when he would act out his issues in session and offer what other analysts have called a "corrective emotional experience"; that is, I would have to behave in such a way as to disconfirm his expectations of people (Alexander, 1963, p. 286). Through my own personal growth, didactic training analysis, and supervision, I would have to monitor my levels of frustration and desire to help. I should not want him to change more than he wants himself to change, for if I do, I am giving him leverage over me, and with ASPs, that is something strongly to be avoided.

9. Are there any areas that you would choose to avoid or not address with this patient? Why?

Given the data I have at the present time, there are no areas per se I would avoid with Frank. As I conceptualize it, it is not an Issue of "areas" as much as it is one of "timing." With any client at all, but with Frank in particular, I would be sensitive to the fact that he may not be ready to hear certain things at certain times. Frank is looking for a fight, and I do not want to fight with him, except in special cases where he might be testing me to see if I'm "tough enough to take it." In those cases, we might butt heads with each other within very narrow and specific guidelines, but only until he can see that I can stand up to him without being intimidated. My goal should never be to defeat him, to make him feel inferior, or to give him the sense that he is "one down" on me. If at any time I believe my work will do just that, I would avoid that area, at least for as long as I could.

10. Is medication warranted for this patient? What effect would you hope/expect the medication to have?

According to the history and testing, there is no indication of mania or a formal thought disorder. A psychiatric and/or neurological consult might prove helpful nonetheless. Some of the newer antidepressants can have potent effects on impulsivity, and possibly anticonvulsant medications could help manage some of his aggression, as might Antabuse help control his drinking. This area is beyond my expertise, however, and that is why I would seek out a consultation. Getting Frank to "have his head examined," though, might prove extremely challenging.

11. What are the strengths of the patient that can be used in the therapy?

Frank has a lot of strengths. He has never quit. Yes, Frank's psychopathology has been difficult for him. It has brought him a great deal of grief, but that grief has been less than what he imagined he would get had he not done the things he did to survive. There is something to admire in his tenacity, stick-to-it-iveness, and power. He served in the military, and he managed to feed himself and those he loved even in tough times.

Frank is here and alive. Given his background, history of abuse, military service, and jail time, he has managed to survive. That is an accomplishment.

He is in therapy. That needs to be acknowledged. Frank doesn't do what he doesn't want to do. I would work hard to reframe his coming in as being a healthy, positive step, not something that he is being coerced into doing.

Finally, he probably has a lot he can teach people, me included.

I have the sense from reviewing the history that rarely has anybody admired Frank or asked him to lead for very long in a non-aggressive context. There probably are many things about leadership, survival skills, and tenacity he could and might even enjoy teaching me (and fellow group members). I would hope to get the chance to have him do that.

12. How would you address limits, boundaries, and limit setting with this patient?

Addressing limits would be a crucial issue with Frank. At the expense of being too clever, a dynamic I know I need to be careful with in such cases, I would need to set limits with Frank in such a way as to not give him a weapon to beat me over the head with. For example, if I make too big an issue of his drinking, he might drink in order to prove he can defeat me. But if I fail to address it at all, he may start coming to session intoxicated. That would benefit no one. One way of addressing such issues might be to have Frank see "them" as "the enemy," and possibly see me as his "ally" in his fight against "them."

As I see it, there are three possible "enemies" we could "attack. First, we could attack his drinking. I would try to reframe his drinking as controlling him, and he being at the mercy of it, and not the other way around. Whereas he sees himself as a "two-fisted drinker," I would want to show him that he may be weak and giving in to the drinking. Toughness would be avoiding the excessive drinking, not managing it.

Next, I would see if we could use the legal system as the "enemy" we have to not let "beat us." (My emphasis upon the "us" IS deliberate.) With the collaboration of the law enforcement personnel, I would try to get Frank to see them as having no faith in him, watching him constantly to see if he'll slip up, and anxiously waiting to embarrass him in public (with only a slight reference to his father's abuse). We would need to do whatever we could to make sure no one ever puts him in such a position again.

Lastly, I would see if I could get some kind of negative response about his father. If my guess is right, Frank is still pretty angry with him. I would attempt to set up his father's style of relating to people as the same way Frank relates to them. By acting like his father, Frank is acknowledging that "that no-good bastard was right." "Frank, you've become just like him. You're paying tribute to him and showing him that you wanted to be just like the way he was. Why would you want to compliment that guy?"

Frank may be a client I would not necessarily sit in my office with and just "talk." We might need to go for walks. Face-to-face conversation might prove too "touchy-feely" for him. Walking along a street outside the office and talking "like two men" might seem more acceptable to him and encourage him to relate to me as someone other than a "doctor" or an authority figure. Maybe it wouldn't; it might simply loosen a boundary that shouldn't be pushed anyway. Nonetheless, I would try it and see if it produced results. If it did not, I would stop.

13. Would you want to involve significant others in the treatment? Would you use out of session work with this patient? What homework would you use?

Besides individual and group psychotherapy, I would use family therapy (Sherman & Dinkmeyer, 1987). He has a wife he cares about. She has been there for him and stuck it out with him. Perhaps his relatives, or at least his brother, would be available. A great deal of negotiation would be needed to have him allow me to bring them in. I would certainly give it a try. His wife might just provide the leverage I need to open him up.

Ideally, if I could bring in many relatives, I would try network therapy. Not just his immediate family, but his aunts, uncles, in-laws, and the like, would be helpful. Adlerians emphasize the social context of problems. Rather than hypothesize what the cost of his style is for those in his social world, I would attempt to actually demonstrate what his style costs him and those around him. Between group and family therapy, Frank might be brought to a point where he would develop common sense.

Many Adlerians find homework invaluable. I do as well. With Frank, I would follow a basic structure that I follow with most of my clients. We would begin each session with a goal, something to learn each session. We would explore it, and try something in session to rectify the problem. Whatever we did in session that seemed to produce a beneficial result would then be assigned as homework between sessions. What he practiced in session would be applied between sessions. Once again, I would have to be careful not to allow myself to be set up for a disappointment. Frank may not want to do much therapeutic work between sessions.

14. What would be the issues to be addressed in termination? How would termination and relapse prevention be structured.

I am not sure what termination would look like with this client. With Frank, clear goals would facilitate compliance, to a degree. ASPs typically do not like too much structure, however; it gives them a sense of being "fenced in," and that they try to avoid. We would need to strike a balance between what is required of him by the law, what is desired of him from his family, what I would like from him as his psychotherapist, and what he wants for himself. In other words, we are back to the beginning, what Adlerians consider the first stage of psychotherapy, goal alignment during the relationship stage. All things being equal, I would like to see him stop or control his drinking, become more empathic, more socially interested, and considerably more flexible in his style. While the fundamentals of his style would probably remain unchanged, he would use his style in a much more constructive manner (Kopp, 1986).

Relapse prevention would entail teaching him about his style of operating and his ability to step outside of his style and catch himself heading down a non-constructive—or destructive—path. For example, Ruling Types are hypersensitive to challenges to their power. We would need to be very concrete about how sensitive he IS to such "affronts" and work with him to become more tolerant of such issues.

With regard to his drinking, we would try to show him the connection between his life-style and his choice of alcohol as a coping mechanism. While there may be dozens of social, economic, organic and environmental reasons people abuse alcohol, Adlerians are interested in the purpose of the abuse (Laskowitz, 1971; Lombardi, 1996). We tend to believe that the substance produces an effect chemically that the individuals feel incapable of producing psychosocially. Frank is a bit of an excitement seeker; it gives him a sense of power and immortality that reinforces the fiction that he is top dog and beyond the limits normal people have. Alcohol may give him a euphoria that makes him feel free. As it lowers his inhibitions, it allows him to try the (sometimes) dangerous things he is about to do. It is "liquid courage," so to speak. Along much the same lines, it will dampen down his emotional responsiveness as well, once he overindulges. This dampening down of feelings after the initial euphoria may help him maintain his apathy, and hence his sense of not caring about anything and therefore being beyond anybody's control. These dynamics need to be explored and more constructive ways of his meeting challenges have to be put in place.

Frank cannot lead a dull life. If his goals of freedom and power are not met in constructive ways, he will "relapse." We would need to find him social activities and a career that would allow him to continue his style, but simply in a more adaptive way.

15. What do you see as the hoped for mechanisms of change for this patient, in order of relative importance?

The hoped for mechanisms of change for this patient would be his ability to be a leader, a fighter, and a survivor. Frank feels inferior, and given his history, this is more than understandable. We would need to target his strengths and encourage them. Rather than ask him to "reinvent himself," we would ask him to realign himself. Whereas in the past he moved towards his goals in a destructive manner, we would ask him to (basically) keep the same style, but use it more·constructively (Kopp, 1986).

REFERENCES

Adler, A. (1956). *The individual psychology of Alfred Adler*. H. L. Ansbacher & R. R. Ansbacher (Eds.). New York: Basic Books.

Adler, A. (1976). Individual psychology and crime. *Journal of Individual Psychology, 32*, 131–144. (Original work published 1930)

Alexander, F. (1963). *Fundamentals of psychoanalysis* (rev. ed.). New York: W.W. Norton.

Beck, A.T., Freeman, A., & Associates. (1990). *Cognitive therapy of personality disorders*. New York: Guilford Press.

Benjamin, L.S. (1996). *Interpersonal diagnosis and treatment of personality disorders* (2nd ed.). New York: Guilford Press.

Dreikurs, R. (1977). *Psychodynamics, psychotherapy and counseling* (rev. ed.). Chicago: Alfred Adler Institute.

Dreikurs, R., Shulman, B.H., & Mosak, H.H. (1984). *Multiple psychotherapy: The use of two therapists with one patient*. Chicago: Alfred Adler Institute.

Hoffman, E. (1994). *The drive for self: Alfred Adler and the founding of Individual Psychology*. New York: Addison-Wesley.

Kopp, R.R. (1986). Styles of striving for significance with and without social interest: An Adlerian typology. *Individual Psychology: The Journal of Adlerian Theory, Research & Practice, 42*, 17–25.

Kopp, R.R. (1995). *Metaphor therapy: Using client-generated metaphors in psychotherapy*. New York: Brunner/Mazel.

Laskowitz, D. (1971). Drug addiction. In A.G. Nikelly (Ed.), *Techniques for behavior change: Applications of Adlerian theory* (pp. 165–175). Springfield, IL: Charles C. Thomas.

Lombardi, D.N. (1996). Antisocial personality disorder and addictions. In L. Sperry & J. Carlson (Eds.), *Psychopathology and psychotherapy: From DSM-IV diagnosis to treatment* (2nd ed., pp. 371–390). Washington, DC: Accelerated Development/ Taylor & Francis.

Maniacci, M.P. (1996). An introduction to brief therapy of the personality disorders. *Individual Psychology: The Journal of Adlerian Theory, Research & Practice, 52*, 158–168.

Maniacci, M.P. (1999). Clinical therapy. In R.E. Watts & J Carlson (Eds.), *Strategies and interventions in counseling and psychotherapy*. Washington, DC: Accelerated Development/Taylor & Francis.

Mosak, H.H. (1995). Adlerian psychotherapy. In R.J. Corsini & D. Wedding (Eds.), *Current psychotherapies* (5th ed., pp. 51–94). Itasca, IL: F.E. Peacock.

Mosak, H.H., & Maniacci, M.P. (1998). *Tactics in counseling and psychotherapy*. Itasca, IL: F.E. Peacock.

Mosak, H.H., & Shulman, B.H. (1967). *Introductory Individual Psychology: A syllabus* (rev. ed.). Chicago: Alfred Adler Institute.

Powers, R.L., & Griffith, J. (1987). *Understanding life-style: The psycho-clarity process*. Chicago: Americas Institute of Adlerian Studies.

Sherman, R., & Dinkmeyer, D. (1987). *Systems of family therapy: An Adlerian integration*. New York: Brunner/Mazel.

Shulman, B.H., & Mosak, H.H. (1988). *Manual for life style assessment*. Washington, DC: Accelerated Development/Taylor & Francis.

Sperry, L., & Mosak, H.H. (1996). Personality disorders. In L. Sperry & J. Carlson (Eds.), *Psychopathology and psychotherapy: From DSM-IV diagnosis to treatment* (2nd ed., pp. 279–335). Washington, DC: Accelerated Development/Taylor & Francis.

CHAPTER 5

Millon's Biosocial-Learning Perspective

Personologic Psychotherapy

Darwin Dorr

I. Please describe your treatment model.

Biosocial-learning theory is a theory of psychopathology and treatment developed by Theodore Millon over 30 years ago (Millon, 1969) in an effort to link current knowledge of personality categories in a logical, deductive manner to existing, acknowledged mental disorders. Biosocial-learning theory is inclusive and anticipated the current integrative approach to personality and psychotherapy (Hubble, Duncan, & Miller, 1999; Norcross, 2002; Norcross & Goldfried, 1992). The amalgam of spheres incorporated in the term "biosocial-learning theory" emphasizes the view that personality and psychopathology develop as a result of the interaction between organismic and environmental forces, an interaction not well-recognized at the time that Millon initially introduced the idea. In his view, this interaction is continuous, beginning at conception and continuing throughout the life cycle. In this way persons who share similar biological/constitutional predispositions may present with differing personality characteristics and clinical syndromes as a function of their experiences. Biological/constitutional factors can shape, facilitate, or limit the nature of the individual's learning and experiences in many ways. Consider, for example, the role of perception. As a result of differing constitutional characteristics persons may perceive the same objective environment in different ways which, in turn, may contribute to marked individual differences in their reaction to the environment. Through this mechanism, the "same" objective environment becomes, in psychological actuality, multiple environments.

Millon does not imply a simple, unidimensional biological determinism in this model. He asserts that biological maturation is dependent upon a favorable environmental experience. The biosocial-learning model posits a circularity of interaction in which dispositions in early childhood evoke counter-reactions from others, which subsequently enhance these dispositions. Children actively interact with their environment, thus contributing to the conditions of their environment which, in a reciprocal manner, provide a template for reinforcement of their biological tendencies.

In 1981 Millon published *Disorders of personality: DSM-III, Axis II,* in which he further delineated and expanded the elements of the personality disorders. In 1990 his *Toward a new personology*, named in honor of Henry Murray and Gardner Murphy's work, extended his theory and incorporated evolutionary principles in personality theory and research. In this book Millon observed that the number and diversity of conceptualizations of personality and psychopathology theory are large and seem to be expanding. Yet the various theoretical frameworks overlap sufficiently to allow the identification of common themes or trends that can be explained by evolutionary theory. He observed that from the early 1900s, therapists repeatedly proposed a three-dimensional structure as a model for describing personality. For example Freud described three polarities that govern all of mental life. Even so, this tripartite model had been identified both earlier and later than Freud in many nations. Millon adopted Freud's polarity model which includes pleasure-pain, active-passive, subject-object. Employing this three-dimensional model as a foundation, Millon described personality patterns that closely approximated each of the Axis II personality disorders in the DSM-IV nosology (American Psychiatric Association, 1994). In the 1990 manuscript Millon was guided by Godel's incompleteness theorem (1931), that no self-contained system can prove its own propositions. Hence, Millon journeyed beyond the parameters of psychology to examine universal principles that can be found in older, more established sciences such as physics, chemistry, and biology. Using the observations gleaned from this broad scientifically historical view, Millon concluded that the principles of evolution are essentially universal and that the lessons to be learned from evolutionary principles have a close correspondence to his earlier (1969) biosocial-learning theory. In updating and revising the theory of polarity, Millon presented the following broad model:

THEORY OF PERSONOLOGIC POLARITIES

Survival Aims:	Pleasure	Pain
	(Life-enhancing)	(Life-preserving)
Adaptive Modes:	Passive	Active
	(Accommodating)	(Modifying)
Replication Strategies:	Self	Other
	(Individuating)	(Nurturing)

In the polyphonic manner of simple Mozartian themes, these polarities can be easily woven into a complex lattice that accurately captures the overarching styles of the various personality disorders. In the case of the antisocial personality disorder, for example, the polarities are out of balance such that the subject's Pain polarity (Preservation) is weak as are the Passive (Accommodation) and Other (Nurturing) polarities. The Pleasure (Enhancement) polarity is average, but the Self (Individuation) and Active (Modification) polarities are strong. Put another way, as a result of the marked imbalance in life's great polarities, the antisocial personality is unmoved by painful consequences, disinclined to conform, and unwilling to sustain or nurture others. On the contrary, the antisocial personality is overly oriented to self and, consequently, diminishes others as a means of securing rewards.

In 1996 the second edition of the Millon's *Disorders of personality* was published together with Roger Davis, which greatly extended and expanded our understanding of Axis II pathology. Millon's 1999 volume, *Personality-guided Therapy*, extended his theory to the practice of integrative psychotherapy which considers the complexities of the whole person.

Millon (1990, 1999) and Millon and Davis (1996) recognized that an integrative theory must consider multiple spheres or domains of personality. Based on a review of the research literature, Millon concluded that it would be clinically useful to focus on eight major domains of personality. Four of these domains are Functional and four are Structural. The four Functional domains are: (1) Expressive Acts, (2) Interpersonal Conduct, (3) Cognitive style, and (4) Regulatory Mechanisms. The four Structural domains are: (1) Self-Image, (2) Object Representations, (3) Morphologic Organization, and (4) Mood/Temperament. Using Millon's system, the practitioner would select one or more of these domains for specific technical interventions at the individual session level. That is, there may be a major deficiency or pathology in one or more of these domains. The clinician would target the deficient domain(s) for specific work in session. In the case of the antisocial personality, Expressive Acts, Interpersonal Behavior, and Regulatory Mechanisms are the domains usually suffering the greatest deficiency.

This approach to treatment is both strategic and tactical in nature. The personologic therapist engages in broad strategic interventions that seek to realign imbalances in polarities as well as in session-based tactical interventions that target deficiencies in specific domains.

Millon also identified what he calls "perpetuating tendencies," that is, characteristics of the personality disorder that actually contribute to the perpetuation of the disorder itself. For example, the overall strategy of the antisocial personality is to "get others before they get me." This defensive strategy naturally provokes counter-hostile reactions on the parts of others, yet the antisocial remains unaware that s/he has contributed to the aggression of others in the first place. Thus, he feels justified in arming himself against further attack. Personologic therapy seeks to identify maladaptive perpetuating tendencies and to counter them where possible.

The system also employs "potentiated pairings" and "catalytic sequences" in mounting a therapeutic program. Potentiated pairings take place when the therapist combines two or more therapeutic procedures simultaneously to overcome problematic characteristics or resistances that might comprise a single approach. Potentiated pairings are selected in a manner that is logically consistent with the theoretical conceptualization of the patient. In the case of the antisocial patient, whose expressive behavior is impulsive, personologic psychotherapy may simultaneously employ the leverage of parole with the influence of family therapy in which family members may be discouraged from being enablers of antisocial behavior.

Catalytic sequences utilize multiple treatment modalities. These are procedures in which serial treatments are applied in an order designed to have the most impact. In the case of the antisocial person, impulsive expressive behavior may first be controlled by legal or other coercive means, after which cognitive approaches are employed to expose errors in thinking. When progress is made in this realm, interpersonal approaches may be used to alleviate difficulties in this sphere.

There are no discrete boundaries between potentiated pairings and catalytic sequences. The idea is that interventions in tandem or sequence may contribute to therapeutic synergy, thus contributing to the effect size. The action of combining interventions is especially important with antisocials because of their notorious resistance to treatment.

At this point it must be emphasized that **Millon's personologic psychotherapy is not yet another "school" of psychotherapy**. Rather, it is a psychological-philosophical model that allows the thoughtful integrationist to conceptualize the assessment and treatment of individuals and to draw a wide variety of therapeutic modalities in mounting the treatment plan. The model is inclusive rather than exclusionary. However, unlike eclecticism, which can be disorganized and haphazard, Millon's personologic therapy provides a theory of psychopathology and a method for directing deliberate interventions logically derived from the model. It affords the clinician a matrix for building a treatment plan based upon logic and thoughtful assessment of the patient's needs, deficiencies, and tendencies. Therapeutic interventions are selected based on the careful conceptualization of the case, not on what one was taught to do in graduate school.

Thus conceptualized, it is unlikely that any legitimate therapeutic approach would be excluded from a personologic therapy plan. However, the clinician would be closely questioned as to why a particular intervention was chosen for a particular client, why the intervention was selected at a particular time in the therapy, and what the strategic or tactical goals and objectives may be for the intervention.

For this reason this chapter will not, by the nature of the system being employed, present a tight description of a particular orthodox approach to the antisocial patient. Rather, there will be an attempt to address the therapeutic issues raised in a manner that is logically consistent with the conceptualizations of the antisocial individual as articulated within the model of personologic therapy.

A final caveat must be offered to the reader. This chapter is being written by an appreciative supporter of Millon's system. However, the interpretation of the system and the notions about interventions for the patient under consideration in this book need not be assumed to be endorsed by Dr. Millon, or for that matter, other adherents to the system. Any misinterpretation or misapplication of Millon's work must be laid at the feet of this writer.

II. What would you consider to be the clinical skills or attributes most essential to successful therapy in your approach?

Personologic therapy provides brief statements about the clinical skills and the attributes of the successful therapist choosing to work with the antisocial patient. Millon and Davis (1996) referred to the work of Beck and Freeman (1990) in this matter. These authors site the attributes of self-assurance, a reliable but not infallible objectivity, a relaxed and non-defensive interpersonal style, a clear sense of personal limits, and a strong sense of humor.

Additionally, personologic psychotherapy acknowledges the importance of common factors in psychotherapy (Dorr, In press). Common factors are those dimensions of the treatment setting (therapist, therapy, client) that are not specific to any particular technique. Considerable research has been compiled on the role of common factors in effective psychotherapy. In their extensive review of the psychotherapy research literature, Lambert and Ogles (2003) concluded that common factors loom large as mediators of treatment outcome. Of relevance to this discussion are the following common factors that have been identified: the therapist as an individual, the therapist's expectation for improvement, the therapist's persuasion with the client, the therapist's warmth and attention, the therapist's understanding, and the therapist's encouragement. Personologic therapy would counsel caution and recommend realistic expectations when working with the antisocial person (as would an adherent to any other approach), but it is characterized by a respect for the power of the common factors to be beneficial to the patient.

Above all else, the personologic psychotherapist must have a broad view of personality, and for that matter, psychology itself. There is little room for dogma in Millon's system. Because persons are so complex, conceptualizations must respect this complexity. Interventions must flow logically from broad and rich formulations of the person. Rigid adherence to a particular conceptualization of psychopathology or to a particular technique would not allow the therapist to access the entire scope of change process that might be utilized with a specific patient. In short, a personologic therapist would likely be high on the characteristic of openness and low on authoritarianism.

As a final note to this section, this writer believes that to be successful with the antisocial individual, one must have some empathy for their often clumsy and frequently transparent methods. In many ways the antisocial is like a wanderer adrift in the cold looking through the window at a warm, loving family enjoying something that he is horribly envious of, and yet does not understand. This, the clinician must understand.

III.

1. What would be your therapeutic goals for this patient? What is the primary goal, the secondary goal, of therapy? Please be as specific as possible

3. What is your conceptualization of this patient's personality, behavior, affective state, and cognitions?

As the Millon system insists that the choice of therapeutic interventions flow directly out of the overall theoretical conceptualization of the patient, these questions III 1 and 3 will be answered in a single section.

In the case of the antisocial personality, the selection of primary and secondary therapeutic goals will be strongly influenced by the clinician's assessment of the severity of pathology found in the patient. Although this is obviously the case in all therapies, the matter of degree of pathology is especially important in the case of antisocial personality disorder because of the widespread belief or observation that many antisocials are untreatable. Hervey Cleckley himself (1941, 1977), who wrote *The Mask of Sanity*, maintained that the psychopath was untreatable. In the nearly 500 pages of Meloy's *The Psychopathic Mind* (1988), only 31 pages are devoted to the matter of treatment and much of this material is devoted to the discussion of the decision when not to treat.

However, should the personologic clinician choose to treat the antisocial, the matter of goals is clear. As is the case with most points of view, personologic therapy recognized that most antisocial persons do not come for treatment voluntarily. In most cases, they come under an ultimatum. In view of the fact that the antisocial person usually does not perceive that he has a problem, the personologic therapist will likely try to impress upon the patient the ways in which his or her behavior is disadvantageous to him or her in the long run. It is recommended that we stand a greater chance of success with the antisocial if he can be convinced that the change might be in his immediate best interest.

In designing a treatment plan for Frank, the clinician should maintain a balance between the overall conceptualization of the person (strategies) and more specific session-based aims (tactics). Viewing the antisocial person as one in whom there is a serious imbalance among the great polarities of life, the personologic therapist would seek to establish some reasonable equivalence between the unbalanced polarities. The personologic conceptualization of Frank is that he is weak on the Preservation, Accommodation, and Nurturance polarities; average on the Enhancement polarity; and strong on the Individuating and Modifying polarities. Accordingly, the therapist would use a strategy which attempts to reduce Frank's almost exclusive emphasis on the self by encouraging Frank to develop a stronger awareness of others who are separate human beings who hold value and are in possession of rights. In time Frank may find an increased sensitivity to the needs and feelings of others as well. The overly active style of extracting rewards by exploiting others would be confronted. The value of flexible accommodation of others would be taught. The therapist may appeal, if necessary, to Frank's overweening self-interest by pointing out that his needs could be fulfilled faster and easier if he were to adopt these attitudes.

Additionally Frank is weak on the life-preserving polarity of the survival aims. This weakness has resulted in physical injury as well as financial and social losses. With this characteristic in mind, the therapist would be to teach him the survival value of moderating his behavior to avoid unnecessary loss.

Another strategic goal which emerges from the conceptualization of the patient would be to counter perpetuating tendencies. In the antisocial, the potential for perpetuating tendencies to cause difficulty is enormous. The pathological elements of the antisocial disorder itself perpetuate its continuance. Frank perceives others as dangerous and untrustworthy, and treats them as such. This behavior provokes like-mindedness in others and evokes their aggressive behavior. The result is that Frank's perception of others as dangerous is continually reinforced, which perpetuates his disorder.

A related perpetuating tendency is Frank's protective shell of anger and resentment. It should be pointed out that this very attitude is the agent provoking the response from others that Frank is so quick to defend against. Equally, it should be pointed out, like the flip side of the coin, that non-defensive, pro-social behavior will be likely to elicit from others a non-defensive pro-social behavior.

At the more immediate tactical level, specific deficiencies in selected domains of personality functioning would be targeted for work during the session. In Frank's profile the primary domain dysfunctions are Expressive Acts, Interpersonal Conduct, and Regulatory Mechanisms. For example, in the Expressive Acts domain, the antisocial is described as impetuous, irresponsible, acting hastily and spontaneously in a restless, spur-of-the-moment kind of manner: he can be counted on to be short-sighted, incautious, and imprudent. He often fails to plan ahead, to consider alternatives, or to heed consequences. It would not be unacceptable to the personologic therapist to utilize external forces to help control Frank's impetuosity, irresponsibility, and restlessness. Legal or domestic restraints may exert external controls that would help compensate and confine these expressive tendencies. Various tactics of limit-setting might be employed as well as cognitive approaches that would help Frank reframe the short-sighted, imprudent tendencies which cause him such difficulty. It might benefit Frank to appraise the thought processes underlying his behavior and the way in which they lead to negative consequences.

The Interpersonal domain is another area of deficiency. Interpersonally, the antisocial is described as untrustworthy, unreliable, and failing to meet or negate personal obligations of a marital, parental, occupational, or financial nature. Antisocial persons actively intrude on and violate the rights of others. They transgress established social codes through deceitful or illicit behavior. Personologic therapy enlists the help of interpersonal therapy to remediate deficiencies in the interpersonal realm. Benjamin (1993) assumes that antisocials have not had a social learning history characterized by warm and nurturing caregivers that might have led to reciprocal warmth and attachment. The interpersonal therapist counters these tendencies with modulated warmth in an attempt to overcome socialization deficits. Great care, however, should be taken not to allow the patient to believe that warmth equates with weakness, as the antisocial will be quick to attempt to exploit the perceived weakness, thus, sabotaging the therapy.

At 48, it is unlikely that Frank is going to be transformed into a warm, loving person by any therapy. However slick the antisocial person appears, he is actually quite clumsy in terms of long-term payoff. Frank's interpersonal episode in the bar illustrates this. His "getting even" resulted in a parole violation and further negative consequences. This might be pointed out to Frank to illustrate how he needs to improve his interpersonal skills, if for no other reason than self-interest. It would have been in his own best interest to have handled the man in the bar differently. He would not be in his current predicament if he had been more accommodating. Hence, the question put to Frank would be, "How could you have handled things differently so that you would not have violated parole?" The value of greater interpersonal accommodation would be emphasized.

The Regulatory Mechanisms domain is also deficient. The primary regulatory mechanism of the antisocial is acting-out. The antisocial is rarely constrained; socially odious impulses are not refashioned in sublimated forms. Instead, they are discharged directly and hastily, usually without guilt or remorse. In psychodynamic terms, the regulatory mechanisms of the antisocial are like primitive defenses such as acting-out, projection, splitting, and primitive denial. The personologic therapist might employ cognitive interventions such as described by Beck and Freeman (1990) in addressing these deficiencies. The therapist may attempt to help Frank understand that "getting even" does not equate with "getting ahead." The futility of the "talon" philosophy may be discussed. That is, Frank may be asked if he wants to "get even" or "get better." He may be taught that long-term gain may be acquired by binding frustration and using it as a source of energy to attain success. A tactical goal would be to help Frank understand that acting out may provide short-lived advantage (e.g., "To get the offending guy off your back!") but that this style has proved to cause him untold travail in the long run. This writer would add that the goals could be described as fostering pro-social thinking and behavior, reducing criminal thinking while increasing pro-social thinking, enhancing empathy, generating control over drives and affect, and promoting postponement of gratification.

To summarize, in Millon's system the therapeutic strategies and tactics for work with the antisocial patient are as follows:

STRATEGIC GOALS
  BALANCE POLARITIES
  • Shift focus more to needs of others
  • Reduce impulsive acting out
  COUNTER PERPETUATING TENDENCIES
  • Reduce tendency to be provocative
  • View affection and cooperation positively
  • Reduce expectancy of danger
TACTICAL MODALITIES
• Offset heedless, shortsighted *behavior*
• Motivate interpersonally responsible conduct
• Alter deviant cognitions

2. What further information would you want to have to assist in structuring this patient's treatment? Are there specific assessment tools you would use (data to be collected)? What would be the rationale for using these tools?

The social history provided is thorough, and it gives a clear picture of Frank's long history of antisocial characteristics. The main thing this writer would like to see is any evidence of pro-social tendencies. As is the case with all personality disorders, antisocial personality is a spectrum disorder. Any island of pro-social tendencies provides a kernel of matter to be nurtured into broader benevolence.

It is not unexpected that a devotee of personologic therapy would be interested in obtaining a Millon Clinical Multiaxial Inventory—Third edition (MCMI—III, Millon, Davis, & Millon, 1997) as it is isomorphic with Millon's theory and largely isomorphic with DSM-IV. Of course an elevation on the Antisocial scale would be expected, but Frank's history makes the question of antisocial personality moot. Of more interest would be any evidence on the MCMI—III of moderating factors. Specifically, it would be of considerable interest to know whether there were any elevations on scales measuring tendencies to internalize. Signs of anxiety, depression, compulsivity, and even somatoform tendencies may indicate some disposition to internalize. Any such tendencies may be moderators with the potential to curb acting-out. Knowledge of such inclinations could help the clinician look beyond Frank's hard-boiled exterior. A disposition to internalize may be used by the therapist to help Frank control his acting-out and thus to achieve a more adaptive and beneficial life style.

Another instrument that would be very useful in combination with the MCMI—III would be the Rorschach, (Exner, 2003). There are many ways in which the Rorschach complements the MCMI—III (Dorr, 1997). The Rorschach is exquisitely sensitive to defects in reality testing. Dorr and Woodhall (1986) found that the reality testing scores of antisocials were equivalent to those of schizophrenics. These subjects had a good capacity to distinguish inner and outer reality and thus the casual observer would not readily infer the depth of disordered thinking. However, antisocials' ability to accurately perceive external events as well as their ability to perceive internal events was compromised. Antisocials rarely presents with psychosis, but they often do present with subtle disorders of thinking. This helps us to understand their convoluted logic. Recall that Cleckley purposely titled his book *The Mask of Sanity,* indicating that the "sanity" was a mask or a veneer of normalcy. In some cases the Rorschach can be very helpful in ruling out schizophrenia, but more commonly, by identifying subtle cognitive quirks that may help us grasp the peculiar logic of the antisocial person.

Many variables on the Rorschach would be of considerable interest, including *Lambda, X-%, Xu%, SUM6, WSUM6, AG, COP, Z-, EA,* and *D* scores. Although Exner (1991, 2003) urges the clinician to use the Comprehensive System as a whole, for the sake of brevity only two variables will be highlighted here. *Lambda* and *X-%* reveal pertinent information about cognitive styles that are very important to the clinician. Antisocials tend to have high *Lambda* scores (Meloy, 1988). *Lambda* provides an index of the degree to which the subject oversimplifies his world to make it less demanding or threatening. A high *Lambda* indicates psychological tunnel vision. It reveals a tendency to avoid, ignore, or reject stimulus complexity as much as possible. It sets the stage for failure to meet the demands of the stimulus situation. According to Exner (1991) a high *Lambda* style may be of considerable interpretative importance. It has significance in terms of overall cognitive style and thus life-style. If Frank's record contained a high *Lambda* score (which it surely must), it would pinpoint a target for intervention. Specifically it would reveal a significant tendency toward cognitive narrowness which may account for many of Frank's difficulties. The therapist may point out to Frank the long-term cost of this cognitive style and work to help him increase his tolerance for complexity and his capacity to rise to the demands of each situation.

A second Rorschach variable that provides important information is the *X-%*. This is an index of the proportion of responses that have bad form and, thus, it yields a measure of perceptual accuracy of the subject. To illustrate the significance of this variable, in profiles given by schizophrenic subjects in Exner's sample, the average *X-%* was 36–38. That is, about 37% of the responses of the schizophrenic patients were of bad form. In contrast, non-clinical adults averaged 7–10% bad form. According to Exner, if the value for *X*-% is in the range of .15 to .20 the clinician should have some concern about the possibility of perceptual inaccuracy and/or mediational distortion. When the value of *X*-% exceeds .20, it is likely that the patient has significant problems that promote perceptual inaccuracy and/or mediational distortion. This indicates that a substantial proportion of these subjects present with perceptual inaccuracy and/or mediational distortion. Deficiencies in information translation contribute to extensive problems in reality testing which, in turn, result in behavior that is inappropriate to the situation. If Frank had a high *X*-%, the clinician would work toward helping him improve the accuracy with which he translates information from the world. If he were not elevated on this dimension we would have a better prognostic sign and we would be able to use his relatively good reality testing as an asset for his recovery.

The Hare Psychopathy Checklist (PCL) (Hare, 1991) may be of considerable utility. The PCL, inspired by Cleckley's original 16 criteria, is based on sound psychological procedures and consists of a 20-item instrument that is rated on a three-point scale. Two correlated factors have emerged from this instrument, a narcissistic variant of psychopathy and a "purer" form of psychopathy. This instrument provides a clear picture of the degree of psychopathy, ranging from mild to severe, and it is very useful in (a) determining the degree of psychopathy and (b) pinpointing specific areas of psychopathic activity. It could be used to rapidly assess the degree of Frank's psychopathic tendencies.

4. What potential pitfalls would you envision in this therapy? What would the difficulties be and what would you envision to be the source of the difficulties?

8. Are their special cautions to be observed in working with this patient (e.g. danger to self or others, transference, countertransference)? Are there any particular resistances you would expect? How would you deal with them?

From the viewpoint of personologic therapy, questions 4 and 8 are highly related; hence they will be addressed in a single section.

The most obvious difficulty, or pitfall, would be the nature of the disorder itself. By its very complexion, the disorder of antisocial personality disorder is resistant to change. The various pathological attributes of the psychopath are egosyntonic. Generally they are proud of their cold-hearted, loner status. In therapy with the antisocial, we are asking him to give up some measure of control, which can lead to anxiety or even panic attack. Because they tend to externalize, antisocials generally feel relatively little psychological discomfort.

As we attempt to encourage them to internalize some discomfort about their behavior, they will naturally be resistant. They will not likely experience the change as positive.

Another obstacle to treatment is what Cleckley (1941) described as "semantic aphasia." The psychopath may be verbally facile in terms of surface language, but the deeper meaning of language is lost. Thus, they can appear to be very cooperative in terms of the words that they emit, but the words may not mean what they appear to mean. The therapist can be duped into believing that real, meaningful change is taking place if the language alone is used as an outcome measure.

Countertransference is a major pitfall in work with the antisocial. Lion (1978) cautions against therapeutic nihilism, a major countertransference issue. Therapeutic nihilism is the belief that antisocials are untreatable. This point of view would assuredly hamper attempts to bring about real cognitive, emotional, and behavioral change. Furthermore, it may lead to a less than objective attitude and even spur a tendency to retaliate against the psychopath.

Fear is another major countertransference problem that can be problematic in at least two ways. First, because therapists tend to think of themselves as benevolent helpers, they may have too little sensitivity to the potential dangerousness of the antisocial and thus place themselves in harm's way. Antisocials can hurt you. Secondly, Meloy (1988) has described the real fear that a clinician can feel in the face of a predatory psychopath. Sensing the danger, the therapist may respond to the veiled or not so veiled threats of the psychopath in such a way as to become immobilized and ineffective.

Meloy also observed that the therapist's fear of being devalued is a countertransference issue. He noted that therapists are sensitive to their patients and generally have a great investment in the patient improving in therapy. The antisocial tends to devalue the therapy and the therapist, and this can lead to a sense of discouragement and devaluation on the part of the therapist. Therapists working with the antisocial had best not be concerned with batting averages.

Regarding the sources of the difficulties mentioned above, all that have been mentioned are inherent in the nature of antisocial psychodynamics. They may also be inherent in the mix between the psychopath and the traditional therapist. To explain further, most therapists go into clinical work to help people who hurt. They do not go into this work to help people who hurt other people. If the therapist does not have a realistic understanding of the nature of psychopathy and what it takes to bring about behavioral, emotional, and cognitive change, little will be accomplished and the potential for harm will increase. The stance taken with the antisocial individual must be considerably different from the stance that one may take with individuals who internalize pain and conflict.

At this point we will turn to special precautions that clinicians should observe when working with this patient. It is obvious that Frank has been a conman all his life, and there is little question that he will try to con the clinician. It is especially troubling that Frank has been adroit at using his anger to intimidate people and that he seems to see this as an acceptable, normal way to control others. He will likely turn to anger as soon as he thinks he is not getting his way with the clinician. A factor that makes this more serious is that he has also used violence to control others, both those known to him and strangers. There is no reason to rule out the possibility that he would be physically violent with the clinician. Even if Frank is not violent, the clinician may find that punches are being pulled out of fear of antagonizing him. This, of course, would lead to poor treatment. Further, it is likely that if the clinician does the job properly, Frank will begin to feel pinned down and out of control. This will anger him, and it is likely that if he cannot displace on the therapist, he will displace on his wife. This should be identified early in therapy, and measures should be taken to ensure her safety.

The issue of anger and violence must be dealt with at the beginning of therapy. It must be made quite clear to him that any inappropriate expression of anger or violence will absolutely not be tolerated and that if this occurs, Frank will be discharged from treatment and the parole officer will be informed of his behavior. The clinician should point out that Frank has been using anger and the threat of violence to get his way all his life and that this has led to many problems. It should be emphasized that this tendency toward anger and violence has caused enormous difficulty in his life, including discharge from good jobs and a prison sentence. The therapist may also indicate that if Frank has any hope of improving his life, he needs to bring these matters under control. Anger and violence should never be tolerated. The clinician should non-defensively emphasize that s/he is not afraid of Frank and that this intimidating behavior has been maladaptive in terms of Frank's purposes in achieving a rewarding life.

Frank is bright, which raises another caution. Despite his inattention to schoolwork he was able to pass his classes, and he was bright enough to become a helicopter pilot. Parenthetically, it is important to emphasize that Frank is likely to be studying the clinician harder than the clinician is studying him. Thus, he is using his intellectual energy in a manner differing from the clinician. The clinician is thinking about the therapy; Frank is thinking about how to beat the therapy. He will use his intellectual energy to calculate how to avoid treatment. The best way to manage this is to confront it in the sessions. The therapist can simply say that Frank is using most of his intellect to con the therapist instead of using his ability to work on the goals and objectives of treatment.

5. To what level of coping, adaptation, or function would you see this patient reaching as an immediate result of therapy? What result would be long-term subsequent to the end of therapy (prognosis for adaptive change)?

The personologic system readily yields information about the prognosis for the antisocial. As with virtually all other perspectives, there is a sense that prognosis is guarded. Millon and Davis (1996) cite Benjamin's interpersonal therapy with the antisocial. Benjamin (1993) cautions that the antisocial cannot enter into a genuine therapeutic alliance with a therapist. She suggests the use of a milieu treatment program in which the antisocial is essentially ignored until s/he begins to comply with the program. At this point the subject gains greater freedom and receives positive feedback from the staff.

In this regard, Millon and Davis (1996) also cite the work of Beck and Freeman (1990). Beck and Freeman emphasize that their model does not try to improve moral and social behavior through induction of shame or anxiety, but rather they employ a cognitive growth strategy to help the patient move from concrete operations to abstract thinking and interpersonal thoughtfulness, that is, into formal operations.

In my own work with antisocials, I tend to emphasize adaptation as opposed to great internal change. I employ a "what's in it for you?" strategy, frequently pointing out the value of complying with social conventions and helping the antisocial to experience gratification in ways that are not dangerous to self or others.

6. What would be your time line (duration) for therapy? What would be the frequency and duration of the sessions?

It is recognized that antisocial personality disorder is generally refractory to change and requires considerable investment of time and energy on the part of the therapist as well as the patient. In my experience with treating patients who are antisocial to any appreciable degree, successful outcomes have always been achieved in long-term work. The work requires that one have some means of external control, such as a prison, parole, or hospital in which the irresponsible acting-out behavior can be dealt with with dispatch. This writer has never observed successful treatment of an antisocial person in six to eight sessions, unless the psychopathic tendencies were very mild and the client was very motivated.

On the other hand, the Millon system recognizes the need for quicker and more efficient therapies. Millon and Davis (1996) assert that by efficiently conceptualizing the difficulties of each of the personality disorders, including the antisocial personality disorder, the treatment may be more efficient than other models. Deficits are quickly identified and the therapy is specifically designed to target these deficits, which might contribute to a shorter duration. Integration of potentiated pairings and/or catalytic sequences together with targeting specific domains may speed the course of therapy.

Although the tendency in the contemporary market is toward shorter therapies, it should be emphasized that the degree of harm that the antisocial visits upon society is enormous. An investment in intensive, long-term therapy may have considerable benefit to society. For example, Yochelson and Samenow (Samenow, 1984) followed up 30 hard-core antisocials who had been receiving long-term treatment in their program. Using a very stringent criterion (not merely that the subjects be free of arrest), 13 of 30 had very few desires to commit crimes. They could account for how they spent their money and time. They not only held jobs; they had developed stable work patterns, and they were advancing. These 13 men represent better than a 33% improvement rate using a stringent improvement criterion. More significantly, each one of these persons represented a one-man crime wave. The savings to society accrued by such a long-term and demanding program are of considerable significance.

7. Are there specific or special techniques that you would implement in the therapy? What would they be?

As noted earlier, personologic approach is not a technique or school of therapy. Rather, it is a way of thinking and conceptualizing the patient's difficulties and using this conceptualization to mount a treatment program. The system would clearly recognize the unique difficulties and challenges posed by the antisocial, and it is open to contributions from a wide variety of therapeutic schools and techniques.

In this section, one technical approach that is compatible with the Millon system will be described. I have used this system for many years with hard-core antisocials with some degree of success. The primary therapeutic technique employed is confrontation (Masterson, 1976). It must be emphasized that confrontation does **not** mean angry attack. Such attempts are fruitless. Technically, confrontation is a therapeutic intervention intended to deal with primitive defenses such as splitting, avoidance, and primitive denial by empathically but intensively bringing pressure on the patient to face the denied maladaptive functioning of these defenses. Confrontation is generally directed at the self-destructive aspects of the patient's life. Confrontation throws a "monkey wrench" into the patient's primitive defense system. Primitive defenses allow the patient to feel good but permit behavior that is maladaptive and harmful to self and others. Confrontation means that the therapist points out the harm the patient is bringing upon him/herself. Thus confronted, the patient finds it more difficult to act out without recognition of the resulting harm. Thus, internal conflict is created where there had previously been none. At this point the therapist can implant the "no pain—no gain" concept which may contribute to forward movement in treatment.

Confrontation is powerful but must be used with great care. The therapist must be really present, empathically in tune with the patient's feeling state. The confrontation must be relevant to the content of the matters being discussed and the patient's patterns of thinking. The confrontation must clearly be in the patient's best interest. Finally, the therapist must confront quietly, firmly, and consistently without being angry or contentious. One must be able to disagree without being disagreeable.

Millon describes the cognitive style of antisocials as "deviant," describing how they construe events and interpret human relationships in accord with unorthodox beliefs. Hence, a cognitive technique that uses confrontation, as defined above, to lead the patient to focus on errors in thinking, is consistent with the model. The specific model used to address errors in thinking was developed by Yochelson and Samenow (1976) in their work with hard-core antisocial persons. The model identifies a large number of errors that pervade thinking of antisocial personalities.

The technical work of this therapeutic approach with psychopaths is relatively more educative than is usually found in traditional psychotherapy. Specific behavioral tendencies and cognitive habits are identified and confronted. The patient must comply with a teaching educational program that requires keeping a log. This serves to increase self-awareness and bring the thinking and behavior into compliance with the therapeutic principles. Samenow (personal communication, 1988) lists 16 tactics which obstruct effective functioning. Examples of some of these variables are as follows: "Builds himself up, while putting others down," "Feeding others what he thinks they want to hear, rather than what they ought to know," "Lying," and "Vagueness." Each of these patterns is identified as they arise in the thinking and behavior of the antisocial. These observations are then used to help the patient understand how these tactics contribute to erroneous thinking which leads to antisocial and sometimes criminal behavior.

Samenow (personal communication, 1988) lists 17 common errors in thinking exhibited in the antisocial and therapeutic responses to these errors.

Four of these are listed below for illustration. The errors are listed in the left column and the recommended therapeutic stance is listed in the right column.

Error	Stance or response of therapist
1. *Victim Stance.* "He started it." "I couldn't help it." "He didn't give me a chance." In general, attempts to blame others.	1. Accept no excuses; bring the focus back to the individual.
2. *"I can't" attitude.* A statement of inability, which is really a statement of refusal.	2. Realize that "I can't" means "I won't" and usually has the reference to doing that which he doesn't feel like doing.
3. *Lack of a concept of injury to others.* Does not stop to think how his actions harm others (except physically): no concept of hurting other's feelings, emotions, anguish.	3. Point out how he is injuring others and ask him whether he would like to be treated this way. Point out that injury is not simply a pool of blood, but that going back on one's word; lying, deceiving others are also injuring others.
4. *Failure to put himself in the place of others.* Little or no empathy unless it is to con someone. Does not consider the impact of his behavior on others.	4. Give him examples of how you do this with him.

In using this technique, the therapist insists that the client keep a log so that the antisocial can track his thinking. One example of work with a young hospitalized antisocial patient may illustrate the use of this technique. The patient was in a hospital specializing in treatment of refractory psychiatric patients of all kinds. He was in an activity therapy group in which the therapist was using a cognitive approach in the manner of Yochelson and Samenow (1976). The group met immediately after lunch. The therapist asked each of the group members to relate what they were thinking about as they walked into the hospital cafeteria to get their lunch just prior to the session. Most people reported thinking about what foods were the most appealing, which ones may be fattening, what other people might be thinking about them, or with whom they might sit. The antisocial patient, having been trained in the procedure being described, explained that he was thinking about the cash register. Specifically, he was thinking that the cash register is where the money was kept. He also was thinking about how the hallway behind the cash register led to a door at the back of the cafeteria kitchen. Outside the door there was a small lawn, and if he ran quickly, he could disappear into the woods behind the hospital. Behind the woods was the expressway. Thus, he was thinking about how easy it would be to take the money from the cash register, slip out the back door, cross the lawn, run through the woods to the expressway, where he could hitch a ride to the next state and abscond with the money.

This illustrates the pattern of thinking of the antisocial. The propensity is almost constant. They think about putting people down, stealing, raping, how to get away with something, how to con the shrink, virtually nonstop. The technique of Yochelson and Samenow (1976) focuses intensely on this kind of thinking and confronts it in order to bring about change.

To return to the above patient, his pattern of thinking was discussed in the group and the negative consequences of the pattern were emphasized, that is, being a psychiatric inpatient, being in jail, being rejected by his parents, etc. The way his thinking differed from that of most of the other people in the group was highlighted. The patient was instructed in ways to identify these errors in thinking and how "cleaner" thinking led to more adaptive behavior and thus to more positive outcomes. The patient was very resistant but follow-up revealed that he did rather well after discharge.

9. Are there areas that you would choose to avoid or not address with this patient? Why?

Generally, it is not fruitful to devote time to reviewing developmental and childhood difficulties. Discussion of the past is usually a waste of time with these persons, and it will likely be used by the patient to excuse or justify present actions. It is more useful to take the position that many people have had unfortunate childhoods, but they do not turn to a life of crime and psychopathic behavior. Developmental and childhood factors should only be used in the context of teaching the patient about his antisocial thinking. The past should only be used to illustrate the long list of criminal and sadistic behavior inflicted on others by the patient.

If the patient begins to show some distress or remorse, it might be legitimate to consider and discuss some early experiences in an attempt to help him come to grips with a sense of loss or depression. However, in the rare event that this does occur, it is usually fleeting, and as soon as the therapist begins to resonate with a patient's difficulties in a more empathic and dynamic way, the patient likely will see this as an opening to remount the attack on disarming the therapist.

It is especially important to stop the patient's storytelling. It is very common for the antisocial to fill up the therapeutic hour with accounts of his daring exploits and adventures as a means of bragging and glorifying the nature of his life. It is also used as a means of intimidating the therapist, who probably leads a much more studious and conventional life, a life that Frank despises.

10. Is medication warranted for this patient? What effect would you hope/expect the medication to have?

According to Sadock and Sadock (2003), 5-hydroxytryptamine (serotonin) has gained attention as a potentially mediating factor in aggression. Rapid declines in serotonin levels or function are associated with increased irritability and, in non-human primates, increased aggression. Some human studies have indicated that 5-hydroxyidoleacetic acid HIAA (5-HIAA, a metabolite of serotonin) levels in cerebral spinal fluid inversely correlate with the frequency of aggression, particularly in persons who have committed suicide. It is for this reason that psychiatrists will sometimes prescribe a serotonin specific reuptake inhibitor (SSRI) to individuals who have some difficulties with aggressive behavior. The hope is that the SSRI may block the reuptake of serotonin in implicated neuropathways, thus increasing the amount of the neurotransmitter available, which may have a mitigating effect on aggression.

Although the diagnosis of cyclothymic or bipolar disorder was not offered in this case, it is clear that Frank has widely fluctuating mood swings, and he can sometimes be extremely high. This is punctuated with irritability, rage, and anhedonia. Sometimes a bipolar or cyclothymic pattern may accompany an enduring personality disorder and there are occasions when psychiatrists may consider the use of some sort of mood stabilizer.

In the case of Frank, however, it is doubtful whether a psychiatrist would consider the use of medication. Indeed, the use of medications might give Frank an opportunity to claim that he has some sort of chemical imbalance which he can use to rationalize his past behavior. More likely, the rages are results of his cognitive view and weak morphologic structure. That is, he thinks of himself as number one, top dog, head man, and when the world does not treat him accordingly, he becomes frustrated and angry. As he has deficient morphologic structure, he has little capacity to bind and/or contain frustration, so he flies into a rage.

11. What are the strengths of the patient that can be used in the therapy?

Frank presents with many strengths that could be used to achieve a prosocial adaptation should he choose this direction. He appears to be intelligent, but he has used his intelligence to con people in a guileless manner. He has good social judgment when he wants to use it, but he uses it to con and delude rather than to better social functioning. His verbal skills seem to be high, but he has used them primarily to evade honest communication. His low anxiety level helps him be courageous, but mostly this was wasted in daredevil activities. It is the therapist's job to help Frank understand that he has squandered his talents. From an evolutionary point of view, Frank's use of his gifts has not been especially adaptive. The position taken by the therapist might be that, at 48 years of age, Frank's style of life has not paid off very well. The goal would be to help him recognize that he would be much further ahead if he used his intelligence, social judgment, verbal skills, and courage more wisely. The therapist needs to paint a picture for Frank of what his life might be if he chooses the straight path.

12. How would you address limits, boundaries, and limit setting with this patient?

As noted earlier, it will be necessary to limit storytelling and off-task behavior in the sessions. Secondly, matters of the therapist's own personal life, including family activities, are off limits. If Frank begins to focus on this, it will be necessary to refocus him on his own difficulties. Boundaries should be carefully established and enforced. This also includes creative alternatives to changing appointment times, number of sessions, starting the sessions on time and stopping them on time. It should be made clear to Frank in the very beginning that if he violates the limits this will be explained to and communicated with the parole officer immediately.

In these cases, a treatment contract may be considered. There are certain pitfalls to a treatment contract because it may call attention to boundaries that the patient can then challenge. On the other hand, firm policies are useful. For example, if the clinician is working in the public sector, the client has the right to treatment but the therapist still has the right to set the conditions of the treatment. If the patient is receiving services in the private sector such matters as payment of fees, starting and stopping time, and relationships outside of the therapeutic frame should be made clear. The policy with regard to dismissal should be explained, that is, whether dismissal occurs after one, two, or three missed sessions. If one is working with an antisocial, it is probably best to be very conservative about the number of missed sessions that will be tolerated.

If the clinician is working with antisocials in a group, the typical process-like group therapy format is generally not used. It is usually better to work with an individual member while the others watch, listen, and try to relate what is going on to their own problems. In most cases, if the therapist permits the other participants to participate they may fall into their predatory stance and try to attack the individual in the "hot seat." Of course, the exception to this is that "it takes one to know one" and the other antisocials in the group may facilitate the confrontation. In general, however, the therapist should carefully control the participation of the other group members.

13. How would you want to involve significant others in the treatment? Would you use out of session work (homework) with this patient? What homework would you use?

The advocate of personologic therapy would be enthusiastic about involving significant others as well as the use of homework because of the belief in opportunistically using potentiated pairings, in which treatment methods are combined simultaneously to overcome resistances that a single interventive strategy may not be able to overcome alone. Combining interventions, or applying them in logical sequence (catalytic sequences), improves the chances for success.

Regarding significant others, the major player would appear to be Frank's wife, Jennifer. It is unclear whether she would wish to participate in Frank's therapy. The brother, Jimmy, might be willing to participate, but again it is unclear if he would be willing. The enlistment of the family can be extremely useful in helping to confront and delimit the antisocial's behavior. Most typically, significant others and family have been conditioned to view the abnormal as normal. They take it as a matter of course that they have been exploited, abused, humiliated, stolen from, lied to, cheated, and verbally or physically abused. Frequently, family members do not realize they have a right to better treatment, and the therapy can be augmented by helping the family members bring themselves to an emotional position in which they will no longer tolerate the bullying, lying, and cheating. It is noteworthy that in many cases individuals who have been abused by the antisocial fail to press charges. It is essential that the antisocial behavior not be excused and that the aggrieved parties should feel free to apply consequences. Often, this is a very important part of therapy.

It is usually very helpful in these cases to educate significant others. Most frequently, they are very puzzled by the nature of the behavior and do not understand psychopathology, much less antisocial pathology. It is useful to teach the family that if they continually find excuses for the antisocial family member, s/he has little chance to improve. The light bulb goes on, so to speak, and as they gain a greater understanding of what is happening they can make natural responses to delimit the behavior in question and to protect themselves. Many families believe that the subject behaves in the way he does because they have done something wrong. Frequently, they feel guilty and have spent thousands of dollars trying to make up for some imagined wrong. Of course, in some cases the families have contributed directly to the psychopathic behavior, in which case this must be confronted. In general, however, this is not the case, and the family needs to be educated about what to expect and how to self-protect.

Homework is also a useful way to combine treatments in order to achieve a greater effect. In the case of the antisocial, assigned homework is especially important. So-called neurotic patients employ the repetition compulsion and do their homework by themselves in between sessions. They think about what has happened and try to find ways in which they can approach a situation differently, etc. Not so with the psychopath. The psychopath simply acts out instead of internalizing and the likelihood that they will do homework on their own is very low.

The homework will consist mostly of logs of antisocial thinking. In Frank's case, it should be made clear that homework is part of the treatment and that failure to complete homework will be reported to the parole officer. If Frank does not turn in his homework, the therapist should make that the subject of the session. The therapist should address the matter in a non-attacking, but confronting manner throughout the session and not let Frank get off the hook.

14. What would be the issues to be addressed in termination? How would termination and relapse prevention be structured?

As a system grounded in evolutionary theory, the Millon system places special emphasis on the adaptational success of the patient. Have the polarity imbalances been balanced? Have self-perpetuating tendencies been controlled? Have deficiencies within specific domains been remediated? And what are the chances that these changes will be maintained?

One of the major goals in termination is to attempt to help Frank realize how positive his life will be if he changes his approach. The positive view of the future must be kept firmly in mind because it keeps the payoff for prosocial thinking and behavior firmly in the mind's eye. Additionally it may be useful to remind him of how bad the past life really was. For example, Samenow (1984) describes the case of "Leroy," a hard-core criminal who benefited from his therapy. Leroy asserted that he no longer wanted a life in which he was always looking over his shoulder for the police.

In the termination, the positive aspects of this new life-style should be emphasized: The fact that the patient has held a job or run a legitimate business, is being straight and honest with other people, is paying bills in a responsible way, and perhaps even building a bank account, that he does not have to be looking over his shoulder anymore playing the antisocial game. All of these should be pointed out time and again as a positive life-style and one in which the antisocial can take great pride.

Relapse is always a possibility. Relapse prevention can be managed by discouraging the antisocial from fraternizing with former antisocial associates who would have a regressive pull on the subject. It is not inadvisable to stretch out the parole for the maximum amount of time to allow the antisocial to use this to control his behavior. In fact, it can be suggested to the antisocial that parole is actually a friendly force which helps him to control his disorder. This way he can develop new habits and he will not have to worry about going to jail or being found out in the future. In the case of Leroy, mentioned above, he put himself "on parole" by continuing to come to his therapist once a week, even after the formal treatment was over, so that he would not become complacent and relapse. He welcomed each review of his thinking in the sessions.

15. What do you see as the hoped for mechanisms of change for this patient, in order of relative importance?

The theoretical mechanisms of change in the personologic system are really no different than those of most approaches to psychotherapy. Millon (1999) acknowledges the role of the common factors, he is aware that technique plays a limited role in the change process, he places great emphasis on the unique personality of the client who is the center of the therapeutic endeavor, and he acknowledges the power of the relationship in helping to foster change. What is different about the personologic system is the way in which it guides the practitioner in conceptualizing the psychological complexity of the individual patient. In *Personality-guided therapy* Millon (1999) wrote:

> . . . the problems our patients bring to us are often an inextricably linked nexus of interpersonal behaviors, cognitive styles, regulatory processes, and so on. They flow through a tangle of feedback loops and serially unfolding concatenations that emerge at different times in dynamic and changing configurations. Each component of these configurations has its role and significance altered by virtue of its place in these continually evolving constellations. In parallel form, so should personality-guided synergistic therapy be conceived as an integrated configuration of strategies and tactics in which each intervention technique is selected not only for its efficacy in resolving particular pathological attributes, but also for its contribution to the overall constellation of treatment procedures of which it is but one" (p. 93,).

Thus, it is not possible to order change factors in order of their potential importance, since each element of the intervention interacts with all others.

Rather, the model acts as a guide regarding how to organize and prioritize the interventions at the strategic (rebalancing polarities) level as well as the tactical level by focusing on deficiencies within the eight domains. As discussed in section III 1 and 3 above, at the strategic level with the antisocial there is an attempt to rebalance polarities and counter perpetuating tendencies. Tactically there is an attempt to offset shortsighted behavior, motivate interpersonally responsible conduct, and alter deviant cognitions.

Millon's personologic model greatly helps the clinician to consider multiple causality and multiple levels of intervention. Within this approach, treatment planning is both broad (strategic) and focused (tactical). Now, of course, most clinicians who favor an integrative approach to treatment strive to consider the complexity of their patient's personalities in their therapy, but the difference is that the personoligic approach provides a model for how to do this in a logical and consistent manner. Eclecticism does not do this for us. Personologic therapy helps us to think broadly and systematically, encouraging us to consider multiple dimensions of the complex persons whom we hope to help.

In personologic psychotherapy, the change process is approached in a balanced manner. On the one hand Millon avoids a mechanistic, "engineering" notion of therapeutic change. He writes,

> Persons are not clay waiting to be passively resculptured. Furthermore, the personality system, functioning as the immune system of the psyche, actively resists the influence of outside forces. To uproot a personality disorder, the clinician must wrangle with the ballast of a lifetime, a development disorder of the entire matrix of the person, produced and perpetuated across the years (1996, p. 173).

On the other hand, he is not sympathetic with totally open-ended classic psychoanalytic models, in which therapy may wander around essentially indefinitely and never reach termination. Millon (1996) asserts,

> We argue that for therapy to be effective, it should be structured and specific enough that something gets done in a planful way, but not so structured and specific that what gets done is not set in stone, regardless of the needs and characteristics of the patient (p. 186).

To summarize, the answer to this important question is that the personologic approach is holistic and the essential mechanisms of change are conceptualized as interactive and synergistic.

ACKNOWLEDGMENTS

I would like to thank Stephanie Tilden Dorr for her editorial assistance in preparing this chapter. I also wish to thank Drs. Theodore Millon and Roger Davis for their thoughtful comments and suggestions regarding the manuscript.

REFERENCES

American Psychiatric Association. (1994). *Diagnostic and statistical manual of mental disorders* (4th ed.). Washington, DC: Author.

Beck, A.T., & Freeman, A. (1990). *Cognitive therapy of personality disorders.* New York: Guilford Press.

Benjamin, L.S. (1993). *Interpersonal treatment of personality disorders.* New York: Guilford Press.

Cleckley, H. (1941). *The mask of sanity.* St. Louis: C.V. Mosby.

Dorr, D. (1997). Clinical integration of the MCMI—III and the Comprehensive System Rorschach. In T. Millon (Ed.), *The Millon inventories.* New York: Guilford Press.

Dorr, D. (in press). The role of common factors in domain-focused psychotherapy for the personality disorders. In S. Strack (Ed.), *Personality and psychopathology.* Hoboken, NJ: John Wiley & Sons.

Dorr, D., & Woodhall, P.K. (1986). Ego dysfunction in psychopathic psychiatric inpatients. In W.H. Reid, D. Dorr, J.I. Walker, & J.W. Bonner (Eds.), *Unmasking the psychopath.* New York: W.W. Norton.

Exner, J.E., Jr. (1991). *The Rorschach: A comprehensive system: Vol. 2. Interpretation* (2nd ed.). New York: Wiley

Exner, J.E., Jr. (2003). *The Rorschach: A comprehensive system: Vol. 1. Basic foundations* (4th ed.). New York: Wiley.

Gödel, K. (1931). *On formally undecidable propositions of principia mathematica and related systems.* Unpublished doctoral dissertation. University of Vienna.

Hare, R.D. (1991). *The Hare Psychopathy Checklist-Revised.* Toronto: Multihealth Systems.

Hubble, M.A., Duncan, B.L., & Miller, S.D. (Eds.). (1999). *The heart and soul of change: What works in therapy.* Washington, DC: American Psychological Association.

Lambert, M.J., & Ogles, B.M. (2003). The efficacy and effectiveness of psychotherapy. In M.J. Lambert (Ed.), *Handbook of psychotherapy and behavior change* (5th ed.). New York: John Wiley & Sons.

Lion, J. (1978). Outpatient treatment of psychopaths. In W. Reid (Ed.), *The psychopath: A comprehensive study of antisocial disorders and behaviors.* New York: Brunner/Mazel.

Masterson, J.F. (1976). *Psychotherapy of the borderline adult.* New York: Brunner/Mazel.

Meloy, J.R. (1988). *The psychopathic mind.* Northvale, NJ: Jason Aronson.

Millon, T. (1969). *Modern psychopathology: A biosocial approach to maladaptive learning and functioning.* Philadelphia: Saunders.

Millon, T. (1981). *Disorders of personality: DSM-III, Axis II.* New York: Wiley.

Millon, T. (1990). *Toward a new personology: An evolutionary model.* New York: Wiley.

Millon, T. (1999). *Personality-guided therapy.* New York: John Wiley & Sons.

Millon, T., & Davis, R. (1996). *Disorders of personality: DSM-IV and beyond* (2nd ed.). New York: Wiley Interscience.

Millon, T., Davis, R., & Millon, C. (1997). *Millon Clinical Multiaxial Inventory—III Manual* (2nd ed.) Minneapolis, MN: National Computer Systems.

Norcross, J.C. (Ed.). (2002). *Psychotherapy relationships that work: Therapist contributions and responsiveness to patients.* Oxford, England: Oxford University Press.

Norcross, J.C., & Goldfried, M.R. (Eds.). (1992). *Handbook of psychotherapy integration.* New York: Basic Books.

Samenow, S.E. (1984). *Inside the criminal mind.* New York: Times Books.

Sadock, B.J., & Sadock, V.A. (2003). *Kaplan & Sadock's synopsis of psychiatry: Behavioral sciences/clinical psychiatry* (9th ed.). Baltimore: Williams & Wilkins.

Yochelson, S., & Samenow, S.E. (1976). *The criminal personality: Volume I; A profile for change.* New York: Jason Aronson.

CHAPTER 6

The Lifestyle Approach to Substance Abuse and Crime

Glenn D. Walters

Author Notes: The assertions and opinions contained herein are the private views of the author and should not be construed as official or as reflecting the views of the Federal Bureau of Prisons or the United States Department of Justice. Correspondence concerning this chapter should be directed to Glenn D. Walters, Psychology Services, FCI-Schuylkill, P. O. Box 700, Minersville, PA 17954-0700.

Frank, the individual whose case was introduced in chapter 2, carries a dual diagnosis of alcohol abuse and antisocial personality disorder and presents with little apparent motivation for change. Some clinicians might be inclined to restrict themselves to one of the three areas (drugs, crime, or motivation) in the belief that a change in one area will automatically mediate a change in the other two areas. However, such an approach assumes the existence of simple causal relationships between the relevant variables. What if the interface between Frank's substance abuse, antisocial behavior, and ambivalence toward change is neither simple nor causal? An overarching theoretical model that addresses all three areas might therefore have a better chance of success than a model that focuses on one variable at a time. To this end, the lifestyle approach to substance abuse and crime is described next.

THE LIFESTYLE MODEL OF CHANGE

The lifestyle model of change is grounded in the overarching integrated-interactive theory of human behavior and development proposed by Walters

(2000b, 2000c). A fundamental tenet of the overarching theory is that evolution has equipped all living organisms with a survival instinct that interacts with a self-altering environment. In posing a threat to survival, environmental change generates tension, imbalance, and fear. The fear response aspires to the highest level of assimilation in humans who have achieved a sense of self separate or distinct from the environment, a perception first observed in human children between the ages of 18 and 24 months (Lewis & Brooks-Gunn, 1979). This response is labeled existential fear. All living organisms devise behavioral strategies to cope with the conflicts that inevitably arise when an organism's life instinct is challenged by a perpetually changing environment. The coping strategies employed by humans are most often cognitive, preventative, and designed to achieve affiliation, control, and status (Walters, 2000b). Hence, people seek social support (affiliation), predictability (control), and a sense of identity (status) as a means of surviving the rigors of a self-altering environment.

The building blocks of the cognitive strategies used to advance a person's life instinct are referred to as schemas (Piaget, 1952). By way of analogy, schemas are to belief systems what neurons are to the central nervous system. A scheme is defined by the overarching theory as a basic unit of meaning drawn from experience and stored in memory. Schemas combine to create schema subnetworks like attributions, outcome expectancies, efficacy expectancies, goals, values, and thinking styles. Schematic subnetworks, in turn, merge to form broader cognitive structures known as belief systems, global beliefs about vital aspects of existence derived from an artificial breakdown of the time-space continuum. The self-view and world-view originate from a dichotomization of the space continuum into events located within the skin (self-view) and events located outside the skin (world-view). The past-, present-, and future-views, on the other hand, evolve from an arbitrary yet conceptually meaningful trichotomization of the time continuum into past, present, and future. The human cognitive system is conceptualized as an amalgam of symbols ranging from the simple and specific (single scheme) to the complex and global (belief system). Table 6.1 provides a brief description of each major schematic subnetwork and core belief system.

It is hypothesized that humans respond to existential fear in one of three ways: despair, patterning, adaptation. Despair is an overincorporative style of interaction marked by high levels of accommodation (modification of an existing scheme to incorporate new information: Piaget, 1952) and a perception of being overwhelmed by change. Because despair arouses unpleasant emotions it is usually not long before it is replaced by patterning or adaptation. Patterning involves repeating a behavior to the point of ignoring

TABLE 6.1
Definitions of Major Schematic Subnetworks and Core Belief Systems

Schematic Category	Definition
Major Schematic Subsystems	
Attributions	Schemas devised to explain one's own or another person's actions.
Outcome Expectancies	Schemas that anticipate the future consequences of a behavior.
Efficacy Expectancies	Schemas that represent confidence in the achievement of a desired end.
Goals	Schematic objectives that guide a person's actions and decisions.
Values	Schematic priorities that shape a person's commitments in life.
Thinking Styles	Distorted patterns of ideation designed to rationalize and support a negative or destructive pattern of behavior.
Core Belief Systems	
Self-View	A person's self-construal, comprised of five parts: reflected appraisals, social comparisons, self-representations, role identity, and possible selves.
World-View	A person's conception of the world organized along four dimensions: organismic-mechanistic, fatalism-agenticism, fairness-inequity, malevolence-benevolence.
Present-View	A person's perception of internal and external stimuli and how he or she acts on this perception, known as the perceptual and executive functions of the present-view, respectively.
Past-View	A person's recollection of the personal and historical past.
Future-View	A person's anticipation of future events and possibilities.

or disregarding the reality of environmental change. To the extent that it produces an illusion of immutability or no-change, patterning is an underincorporative style marked by high levels of assimilation (incorporating new information into an existing scheme: Piaget) and low levels of accommodation. Whereas despair and patterning entail hypersensitivity or insensitivity to environmental events and overflexibility or rigidity in the face of change, adaptation embodies moderate levels of sensitivity and flexibility and blends assimilation and accommodation into a single response. Accordingly, adaptation better serves the goal of survival than either despair or patterning.

Patterns or habits are universal human phenomena, but when they become a significant source of affiliation, predictability, and status for an individual they are more properly labeled lifestyles. The overarching theory identifies four families of lifestyle based on the intersection of two anthropologically relevant dimensions: dominance-submission and high-low control. One of the four families, the rebel line (dominant-low control), covers two lifestyles

TABLE 6.2
The Eight Thinking Styles Associated with the Drug and Criminal Lifestyles

Mollification	Making excuses and blaming others for the negative consequences of one's actions. Involves a clear pattern of externalizing responsibility. Ex.: "I wouldn't need to drink if my wife wasn't always bitching."
Cutoff	Rapid elimination of common deterrents to crime, drug use, and other irresponsible behavior. The most common expression of the cutoff is the two-word phrase "fuck it." Ex.: "I'm not putting up with this crap any longer; I'm going in to see the boss right now and tell him I quit!"
Entitlement	A sense of ownership or privilege designed to give one permission to use drugs or engage in criminal behavior. Entitlement is often marked by the misidentification of wants as needs. Ex.: "I need to steal in order to support my drug habit; after all I am addicted."
Power Orientation	The desire for control over others. Within the drug lifestyle a unique expression of the power orientation is the desire to gain control over one's emotional state through the use of chemicals. Ex.: "Don't mess with me; I'll show you the meaning of respect!"
Sentimentality	Doing something nice for another person in a self-serving effort to feel better about oneself. Ex.: "Selling drugs is no big deal; after all, don't I deliver turkeys to everyone in the neighborhood each Thanksgiving?"
Superoptimism	Believing that one can continue engaging in a negative pattern of behavior without suffering the natural negative consequences of that behavior. Ex.: "I'm not hooked on drugs; I can stop any time I want."
Cognitive Indolence	Rather than dealing with a problem or issue, directly taking a short-cut that critical analysis demonstrates will eventually lead to failure. Ex.: "As soon as I start drinking all my problems seem to disappear."
Discontinuity	Lack of consistency or follow-through in one's thinking and actions. Person is easily side-tracked by environmental distractions and temptations. Ex.: "Every time I leave prison I start out with good intentions, but it is only a matter of time before I am back to using drugs and committing crime to support my habit."

with which Frank is well-acquainted. To the extent that the drug and criminal lifestyles fall into the rebel class of lifestyles they exhibit similar patterns of interaction and are supported by a common set of beliefs or thinking styles. The eight thinking styles that the drug and criminal lifestyles share in common are listed in Table 6.2. Several of these thinking styles (cutoff, sentimentality, superoptimism) stem from Yochelson and Samenow's (1976) work on the criminal personality. These thinking styles are not construed as personality traits but as features of a person's ongoing interaction with the environment. Like the environment, thinking styles are continually being altered in response to new situations and experiences and each lifestyle and thinking style assumes a distinctive pattern of interaction with the environment.

Outside of the existential conditions into which people are born, namely a biological organism whose very survival depends on how he or she interacts with a constantly changing environment, people construct their own realities and go about defending these realities. Change, therefore, is principally designed to alter one's perception of reality as manifest in the belief systems to which one subscribes. The overarching theory takes notice of the fact that many more people exit a drug (Walters, 2000d) or criminal (Shover, 1996) lifestyle spontaneously, in other words, without professional assistance, than improve through formal treatment. In fact, the lifestyle approach rejects the medical model of treatment in favor of a procedure whereby the counselor or therapist, known generically as the helper, is tasked with facilitating the natural change process believed to exist in all people. Stimulating this universal process requires a helper who can focus the client's attention on what are commonly referred to by lifestyle therapists as the four key elements of change: responsibility, confidence, meaning, and community. Accepting responsibility for the consequences of one's actions, possessing skills that improve one's odds of success, finding new meaning in life, and appreciating the impact of one's behavior on the community in which one functions are accorded a central position in the lifestyle theory of change.

ESSENTIAL CLINICAL SKILLS

As an integrated paradigm, the lifestyle model of change borrows extensively from traditional schools of psychotherapeutic endeavor. Out of the psychodynamic tradition comes lifestyle theory's emphasis on the therapeutic relationship. The shaman effect, the psychological equivalent of the placebo effect, is the means by which a therapeutic alliance is forged with clients enrolled in a program of lifestyle change (Walters, 2001). Five factors contribute to the shaman effect: sensitivity, ritual, metaphor, dialectics, and the attribution triad. In the case of sensitivity, the client perceives that the helper comprehends his or her inner world and can assist in rearranging this world. Growth-promoting rituals must replace drug- and crime-based compulsions and metaphors must be invented to construct a shared private meaning between helper and client. Identifying counter-myths to a client's personal myths and forming a synthesis of the two by way of the dialectic method can go a long way toward fostering adaptability. Finally, the three components of the attribution triad (belief in the necessity of change, belief in the possibility of change, belief in one's ability to effect change) impart responsibility, hope, and confidence, respectively, by way of the evolving therapeutic relationship.

In line with traditional behavioral models, the lifestyle approach pays homage to skill development. Learning to manage the internal and external conditions that surface in support of a drug or criminal lifestyle is critical if change is to occur. Clients may be taught relaxation and stress manage-ment skills to alleviate powerful feelings of existential fear and they can be trained in access reduction to limit their exposure to drug- and crime-related cues and opportunities. Clients can also learn how to make better choices. As such, the helper needs to be well-versed in techniques that boost client confidence and enhance the client's capacity for sound judgment and deci-sion-making. A third group of techniques capable of championing change in people aligned with a drug or criminal lifestyle is the cognitive and rational restructuring strategies that have become so popular in psychology over the past several decades. Helpers capable of instructing clients in how to use the cognitive models of Albert Ellis (Ellis & Dryden, 1997) and Aaron Beck (Beck, Wright, Newman, & Liese, 1993) to identify and correct irrational and erroneous thinking are an asset to any program of assisted change operating under the lifestyle banner.

The lifestyle approach also borrows extensively from the existential and humanistic traditions in the sense that freedom, responsibility, and mean-ing are stressed throughout the intervention process. Gains initially achieved through the therapeutic alliance (shaman effect) and early skill development (condition-based, choice-based, and cognition-based skill building) can be solidified by instructing the client to alter his or her involvements, com-mitments, and identifications. Involvements change when the client begins performing activities incompatible with crime and drug use and starts associ-ating with people outside these lifestyles. A change in commitment connotes that new priorities, values, and expectancies have replaced old drug- and crime-based priorities, values, and expectancies. Identifications are altered when a client forms a new identity uncontaminated by previous drug and criminal attachments. Avoiding labels formerly ascribed to the client, that is, option-limiting attributions like criminal, hustler, alcoholic, and addict, is one way a person can alter his or her identifications. Helpers working with the lifestyle format are encouraged to emphasize these maintenance strategies in their work with clients.

SPECIFIC QUESTIONS

1. Therapeutic goals

The lifestyle approach reframes and reorganizes primary and secondary therapeutic goals into short- and long-term objectives for intervention. Two short-term objectives in working with someone like Frank are to help him realize that a problem exists and to encourage him to take greater personal responsibility for resolving the problem. Frank is faced with the prospect of returning to prison should his parole be revoked on charges of drunk and disorderly conduct. Confronting him with the negative consequences of his alcohol abuse and criminal behavior may afford him the opportunity to learn from his past mistakes. Some psychologists may label Frank a psychopath and assume, on the basis of this diagnosis, that he is incapable of learning from the consequences of his actions because of inadequate autonomic arousal (Hare, 1993). In some cases, however, the person may have never learned how to profit from these naturally occurring life lessons. Frank's legal predicament has the power to modify his thinking and behavior should he perceive it as a crisis. A crisis is the perception that a lifestyle, in this case an amalgam of the drug and criminal lifestyles, is currently generating more pain than pleasure. By taking naturally occurring events in a person's life, such as Frank's legal predicament and the strain his actions have placed on his marriage, it may be possible to initiate and develop a crisis of sufficient magnitude to temporarily arrest lifestyle activities.

Temporary cessation of lifestyle activities allows people the opportunity to alter the belief systems that may be reinforcing and maintaining their lifestyle. This is the point at which short- and long-term therapeutic goals intersect, the latter of which can be organized according to the four key elements of change: responsibility, confidence, meaning, and community. With respect to responsibility the long-term goal is to help Frank start accepting responsibility for his actions and stop blaming others for the negative consequences of his bad decisions. Confidence is achieved with skill development, which in Frank's case might entail showing him how to reduce the harm associated with his use of alcohol, cope with stress in ways other than drinking, and solve the problems of everyday life without resorting to crime or alcohol abuse. Frank's meaning in life is encapsulated in his self- and world-views, both of which will need to be modified if he is to change his criminal and drug-using behavior. The long-term community goal with someone like Frank is to help him appreciate the negative impact his drinking and antisocial conduct are having on the handful of people who remain in his life.

My guess is that Frank will initially attempt to ingratiate himself to the helper and that, once he realizes that he cannot charm or bully his way out of his predicament, his demeanor will quickly change to one of anger and indignation. Imploring the helper to acquire an intimate knowledge of the client's personal reality does not mean that the helper necessarily endorses that reality. Just the same, the helper must negotiate the difficult task of entering a client's inner world of belief systems without losing his or her own sense of reality, which, it should be noted, is just as subjective as the client's. To this end the helper is encouraged to form a therapeutic alliance with the client and remind the client of the negative long-term repercussions of a faulty alliance. In Frank's case one such consequence is reincarceration. Overtures for cooperation can be sheathed in the logic that working together supplies Frank with the best chance of avoiding jail. Of course, incarceration itself is a life lesson. Pinpointing naturally occurring crises in Frank's marital relationship and economic situation is another way to boost his motivation for change. Once the short-term goal of motivation for change is realized, long-term goals for increased responsibility, confidence, meaning, and community can be implemented.

2. Further information.

There are four measures that would be of considerable assistance in working up a plan of intervention for someone like Frank. First, the Lifestyle Criminality Screening Form (LCSF: Walters, White, & Denney, 1991) and Drug Lifestyle Screening Interview (DLSI: Walters, 1994) are brief assessment tools that produce scores useful in gauging a person's degree of involvement in a criminal and drug lifestyle, respectively. The LCSF is a chart audit form that appraises the four interactive styles of a criminal lifestyle (i.e., irresponsibility, self-indulgence, interpersonal intrusiveness, social rule breaking) and generates an overall score that can range between 0 and 22. From the limited information provided in the case history, Frank should receive a score of at least 10 (the traditional cutoff score for significant involvement in a criminal lifestyle) on the LCSF. The DLSI is a brief structured interview designed to assess the four interactive styles associated with a drug lifestyle (i.e., irresponsibility/pseudresponsibility, stress-coping imbalance, interpersonal triviality, social rule breaking/bending). Since the DLSI follows an interview format, there is no way to know how Frank would have scored on this measure, though data from the case history (early onset of drinking, aggressiveness while drunk, shrinking circle of friends) denote that Frank may be as invested in a drug lifestyle as he is in a criminal lifestyle.

Two other psychological instruments potentially capable of shedding light on Frank's position vis-à-vis the drug and criminal lifestyles are the Psychological Inventory of Drug-Based Thinking Styles (PIDTS: Walters & Willoughby, 2000) and the Psychological Inventory of Criminal Thinking Styles (PICTS: Walters, 1995). Both instruments consist of 80 items designed to measure the eight thinking styles presumed to support a drug (PIDTS) or criminal (PICTS) lifestyle (mollification, cutoff, entitlement, power orientation, sentimentality, superoptimism, cognitive indolence, discontinuity). Given that estimated scores on the DLSI and LCSF insinuate that Frank is involved in both a drug and criminal lifestyle, it would be appropriate to administer both the PIDTS and PICTS, although experience has shown that the two inventories often produce similar results in the same person (Walters, 1998a). From what was written about Frank in the case history, it is speculated that he would likely achieve elevated scores on the mollification (externalization of blame), cutoff (alcohol and violence), and power orientation (desire for control over others through violence and over one's own affective state through alcohol) scales of the PICTS/PIDTS. Understanding how these three thinking styles protect Frank's drug and criminal lifestyles could go a long way towards clarifying his actions and buttressing his overall life adjustment.

3. Conceptualization of personality, behavior, affective states, and cognitions.

Lifestyle theory does not ascribe to a personality view of behavior despite the obvious parallels between Frank's symptoms and Cleckley's (1941/1976) core characteristics of psychopathy. Instead, Frank's symptoms are ascribed to an environment by temperament, interaction (high activity level, low positive emotionality, high negative emotionality, low sociability, high information processing speed, moderately high novelty-seeking), the outcome of which reveals an individual best described as active, bright, unemotional, and socially superficial. What are viewed as traits by most personality theorists are conceptualized as interactive styles and belief systems by those affiliated with the lifestyle perspective. Several of the schematic subnetworks that have evolved from interactions between Frank's temperament and various environmental circumstances include blaming attributions, strong positive and weak negative outcome expectancies for alcohol and crime, high self-efficacy for crime but low self-efficacy for prosocial behaviors, goals that are short-term, values that are hedonistic, and dependence on thinking styles like mollification, cutoff, and power orientation.

The self-view is modularly organized and broken down into five principal components: reflected appraisals, social comparisons, self-representations, role identities, and possible selves. Reflected appraisals are how a person believes he or she is perceived by others. An example from Frank's life would be his reflected appraisal as a bully. Social comparisons can be upward, downward, or parallel for the purposes of self-advancement, self-enhancement, and self-evaluation, respectively. Frank's self-view is dominated by downward comparisons to the extent that he considers himself superior to others and is customarily condescending in his interactions with others. Personal characteristics and features of the environment with which a person identifies are known as self-representations. The self-representations that mark Frank's self-view center around power and control, as epitomized by his muscular build and suspected fascination with firearms. Role identities are the social roles from which a person gains a sense of identity. A principal role identity for Frank, albeit one over which he demonstrates a fair amount of ambivalence, is his prior role identity as a helicopter pilot in Viet Nam. Possible selves are normally divided into desired selves (what I want to be) and feared selves (what I don't want to be). Frank's father served as both a desired self and a feared self for Frank. He craved his father's power but resented his abusiveness. Just the same, he incorporated both possible selves into his self-view.

Whereas the self-view is organized into modules, the world-view is organized into dimensions. Like many who function within the broad parameters of a criminal lifestyle, Frank clearly favors the mechanistic pole of the organismic-mechanistic world-view dimension. In fact, Frank's propensity to manipulate and conceive of the world as a giant chessboard can be traced back to his mechanistic world-view. Fatalism also figures prominently in Frank's world-view. He denies that his drinking is causing him problems and seems resigned to the fact that it is his destiny to be misunderstood and picked on. Frank manifests a schism on the fairness-inequity dimension of his world-view. While he believes that other people get what they deserve and has little compassion for their plight (fairness), he believes that he himself has been victimized by injustice and deserves more out of life than he has thus far received (inequity). Frank's world-view emphasizes the malevolent pole of the malevolence-benevolence dimension and as such he often attributes other people's actions to malicious motives and evil intent.

The three time-based belief systems, the present-view, the past-view, and the future-view, may shed as much light on Frank's conduct as his self- and world-views. The present-view is organized functionally and encompasses two primary functions, a perceptual function and an executive function. Everyone distorts their perception in order to make their experience more compatible with their belief systems and personal sense of reality. For Frank, distortion is part and parcel of his belief systems, at least where the present-view is concerned. Despite above-average intelligence, the executive function of Frank's present-view is visibly impoverished, which in turn impairs his judgment. As is often observed in people who abuse drugs and commit crime, Frank's past-view is negatively valenced. His recollections of the past, from his childhood to his experiences in Viet Nam, are tinged with themes of death, injustice, and betrayal, whereas the more positive aspects of these experiences are largely inaccessible to recall. The one notable exception to this rule is the euphoric recall that Frank has for alcohol and crime, in which the positive aspects of his encounters with drugs and crimes are accentuated and the negative aspects minimized. The anticipations that comprise Frank's future-view portray drug and criminal motifs, plots that he plans to hatch in the not-too-distant future, as exemplified by thoughts of expanding his chop shop operation and taking bets from compulsive gamblers.

4. Pitfalls in therapy.

One potential pitfall for anyone entering into a therapeutic relationship with Frank is his manipulativeness. The record reflects that Frank is adept at identifying and capitalizing on a person's weaknesses. Should he find that he cannot bully the helper into submission he will seek to subtly manipulate him or her by assuming the role of a perfect patient. Lifestyle interventions are often conducted in groups of similarly disposed members. Under such circumstances Frank may try to assume the role of a junior therapist, pointing out the thinking errors and lifestyle patterns of fellow members without volunteering much information about himself. There are perils in working with a client like Frank, whether the sessions are conducted individually or in group, and proper precautions need to be taken. To guard against being drawn into one of Frank's manipulations, the helper should verify Frank's self-report against information gathered from his wife and parole officer while maintaining the confidentiality of his or her conversations with Frank. Trust is a cardinal feature of the therapeutic alliance but it builds slowly when working with someone as deceptive as Frank. Anyone working with Frank in therapy or counseling would be naive to ignore his manipulative manner, yet this awareness should not prevent the helper from entering fully into a productive working alliance with Frank, enlisting the shaman effect, and encouraging Frank to be mindful of the four key elements of change (responsibility, confidence, meaning, community) in his daily interactions with others.

A second trap that could ensnare a well-meaning professional is the belief that either drinking or crime is the principal cause of Frank's difficulties and that altering the "causal" factor will automatically change the "effect" variable. The relationship between drugs and crime, however, is formidably complex. In some instances crime is the principal cause of drug abuse and in other instances drug abuse is the primary cause of crime, but in the vast majority of cases crime and drug abuse coevolve to where they are either reciprocally related or causally independent of one another (Walters, 1998a). In any event, both lifestyles typically need to be addressed. The advantage of the lifestyle model is that it furnishes a philosophy and mechanism by which the two lifestyles that govern Frank's behavior can be examined concurrently, since they are assumed to derive from the same family of lifestyles (rebel) and are believed to share many of the same interactive patterns, belief systems, and thinking styles. Hence, the lifestyle approach is prepared to tackle the drug and criminal lifestyles simultaneously rather than sequentially, which in the long run provides a more cost-effective and coordinated intervention. For instance, cues that trigger crime and drug use (friends, feelings, and situations) are often related if not identical. The pitfall of covering only part of the problem can be rectified by using the lifestyle procedure in which both parts of the problem are included in the solution.

5. Prognosis.

Clinically, helping clients elevate their level of adaptive functioning is the ultimate goal of lifestyle intervention. Whether or not clients expand their adaptive resources depends to a large extent on their ability to realize the four key elements of change described earlier in this chapter: responsibility, confidence, meaning, and community. With or without professional assistance, seeing a spontaneous remission is more common than intervention-related change in persons who have successfully abandoned a drug or criminal lifestyle (Walters, 1998a, 2000d). The key to change is becoming more responsible, confident, purposeful, and community-minded. Frank will present a challenge no matter what model the therapist operates out of because he does not view himself as having a problem. A strong therapeutic alliance is consequently required to combat Frank's fervent defensiveness and the best way to achieve such an alliance is to encourage development of the shaman effect. In fact, the therapeutic alliance is considered central to any intervention designed to improve a client's adaptive capacity.

6. Time line for therapy and frequency and duration of sessions.

The lifestyle approach makes liberal use of group intervention and therefore Frank would likely be seen individually at first and then group therapy would assume increased importance as the intervention proceeded. I have observed in my own clinical work with substance abusing offenders that other persons who have lived these lifestyles are often better sources of encouragement and confrontation than professionally trained therapists who have never lived the lifestyle. In the drug treatment field it is not uncommon for programs to hire paraprofessionals who are "in recovery" themselves in an attempt to make the intervention more relevant. An even better option may be to arrange for professionally trained helpers to supervise groups of parallel lifestyle participants who are at different phases of the change process, so that the confrontation comes principally from fellow group members rather than from the therapist. There is every likelihood that Frank will attempt to manipulate the individual and group sessions, but he is more apt to hear corrective feedback that impacts on his belief systems from peers in a group session than from the therapist in an individual session. Given that it will take several months to form a working therapeutic alliance with Frank, it is anticipated that a minimum of 6 months and a maximum of 2 years (1 hour of individual counseling and 90 minutes of group per week, with the individual sessions slowly being faded out) may be required to stimulate the natural change process which at the present time lies dormant in Frank.

7. Specific or special techniques.

Skills training is an integral part of the lifestyle intervention process, not only for the purpose of instilling confidence but also as a way of promoting responsibility, meaning, and community. One area of skills training that bears directly on Frank's drinking is the possibility of instructing him in the controlled use of alcohol. For reasons delineated in question 9, Frank is probably not going to relate to the abstinence philosophy espoused by Alcoholics Anonymous. Skills-based alternatives like controlled drinking and harm reduction should accordingly be entertained. Research indicates that it is possible to train heavy drinkers like Frank to monitor and control their alcohol intake to the point where it no longer interferes with their daily functioning (Walters, 2000a). Harm reduction in which such high-risk practices as heavy intoxication and drunk driving are targeted for elimination yet alcohol use itself is not banned has been found to be both popular and effective with younger drinkers (Marlatt, Larimer, Baer, & Quigley, 1993). The primary issue with respect to Frank's drinking is helping him to objectively evaluate the impact of alcohol on his health, marriage, and freedom and then draw up a plan that addresses these problems while taking into account Frank's feelings on the subject. Decreeing that Frank never drink again given his present state of mind will accomplish little more than further provoke his resistance to moderation.

Other skills-based approaches could be implemented to augment Frank's adaptive skills and limit his dependence on the drug and criminal lifestyles. Framing intervention as the means by which the four key elements of change are conveyed to clients may be one way of loosening the hold the drug and criminal lifestyles have on Frank. Problem-solving training, for instance, may encourage responsible behavior through improved decision-making ability. Confidence could be enhanced with the aid of procedures that help Frank cope more effectively with negative affect. Techniques designed to teach basic anger and stress management skills like assertiveness training and relaxation training may be particularly effective in assisting Frank in the management of negative affect. Frank's meaning can be reshaped by procedures that expose the irrational roots of his world-view to the light of reason. Rational emotive therapy (Ellis & Dryden, 1997) and cognitive restructuring (Beck et al., 1993) can be particularly helpful in this regard. Community or social interest could be nurtured with a simple procedure that has been around for 80 years (Adler, 1973). A helper employing Adler's simple technique might ask Frank to list three things he can do to help out his wife. It should be noted that while various therapeutic techniques can facilitate the natural change process, lifestyle intervention is attitude- rather than technique-driven, and that none of the techniques described in this procedure will prove effective in the absence of a solid therapeutic alliance.

8. Special precautions.

It is reasoned that because of a high degree of self-centeredness Frank is at low risk for suicide at the present time. Furthermore, his tendency to externalize blame for problems that he himself invites suggests that he probably presents a greater danger to others than he does to himself. Nonetheless, it would not be outside the realm of possibility for Frank to threaten self-injury or engage in superficial suicide gestures in a manipulate ploy to win sympathy or gain concessions. There is also the remote possibility that if Frank abandons his externalization defenses and starts accepting responsibility for his actions, he might eventually become suicidal as he begins to experience the pain he has caused others. This possibility is made even more remote by the lifestyle practice of stressing confidence and community along with responsibility in intervening with clients. Of greater concern than self-injury is Frank's propensity for violence and the threat he poses to others, particularly his wife. Given the fact that Frank's wife has participated actively in the data-gathering phase of the evaluation it is likely that he harbors significant antipathy toward her. She needs to be counseled with respect to her right to protection from abuse and could perhaps benefit from a referral to another psychologist who might be able to work with her on issues of self-esteem and assertiveness.

Being a relationship-based model of intervention, lifestyle theory takes such phenomena as transference and countertransference seriously. All the same, unlike psychodynamic theory where transference and countertransference are attributed to unconscious motives, the lifestyle approach ascribes transference and countertransference to instances where information from the past-view filters into the present-view. Whereas most people are not fully cognizant of the roots of their transference reactions, the process is not viewed as unconscious in a Freudian sense. The transference reactions that are anticipated with Frank are those that center around his beliefs about his father, who was apparently highly abusive toward Frank and his brother as they were growing up. As so often happens in families, Frank and his brother responded differently to their father's abuse. Frank's brother cried, while Frank became stoic. In identifying with the aggressor Frank adopted many of his father's mannerisms and bad habits. Frank's thoughts and feelings towards his father need to be addressed within the context of the client-helper relationship. Projecting blame onto others for problems that he has caused and fatalistically believing that aggression and violence are his destiny must also be challenged. According to information provided in the case history, Frank has mastered the art of identifying people's weaknesses and using this information against them. Self-understanding on the part of the helper is the best protection against a client who tries to kindle a countertransference reaction in an effort to sabotage the therapy to which he has been remanded.

In the opening series of evaluations Frank displayed a marked degree of resistance and uncooperativeness. Rather than adopting the position that Frank is unmotivated toward change, an alternative view, and the one adopted by lifestyle theory, is that Frank is ambivalent toward change (Miller, 1985). Change and continuity are considered the cornerstones of adaptive living. Too much change and the organism feels unstable and stressed; too much continuity and the organism becomes stagnant. The dynamic interplay of these two opposing forces is the source of adaptation. Throughout his life Frank has chosen continuity over change, resulting in prolonged periods of lifestyle adjustment punctuated by brief episodes of extreme stress when the consequences of his lifestyle have caught up with him. This has fostered within Frank a pronounced fear of change. What Frank needs to understand is that change is as natural as breathing and that to ignore change is tantamount to holding one's breath in the belief that air is unnecessary for survival. Guided by the unfolding therapeutic alliance, Frank will be encouraged to reevaluate his old beliefs and construct a new perspective in which environmental change is viewed to be one of the few concrete realities in the phenomenologically informed theory proposed by Walters (2000b, 2000c). Ironically, the therapeutic relationship is both a cause and principal solution for client resistance and is more likely to fulfill the latter function once the helper gains a sense of the client's phenomenological world and shares this knowledge with the client.

9. Topics to avoid.

There are no topics, subjects, or areas that should be off limits in therapy. I may not agree with a client's views on a particular subject but the client has the right to air these views. When conducting a lifestyle intervention the helper follows the client's lead, and if beliefs and goals antagonistic to the helper's value system surface (e.g., Frank wants to learn how to avoid feeling guilty after beating his wife), they are addressed immediately in an honest and straight-forward manner. Although there are no topics, subjects, or areas that are off limits in therapy there are some procedures and techniques that may be largely ineffective with Frank. The 12-step approach used by Alcoholics Anonymous (AA) is one such example. Attributions of personal powerlessness and efficacy expectancies tied to a higher power will probably not sit well with Frank, who is not about to surrender personal control to something outside himself. Whereas Frank should not be discouraged from seeking help from programs like AA, there is a good chance of him joining the parade of first-time attendees who never return for a second meeting. Rather than branding Frank and the mass of other substance abusers who cannot identify with or accept the philosophy and procedures of AA as being addicts in denial, we need to entertain alternative explanations and interventions. The lifestyle model is one such alternative in which the emphasis is on empowerment and self-reliance rather than powerlessness and other-dependence.

10. Use of medication.

The lifestyle approach is an anti-medical model but not anti-medication. In clients suffering from serious mental disorders of known biological origin (e.g., schizophrenia, bipolar disorder, major depression, obsessive-compulsive disorder) the intervention of choice is often medication and the individual needs to be referred to a psychiatrist for evaluation to determine the type and dosage of psychotropic medication required to provide symptom relief. Frank, however, does not satisfy the criteria for any of these disorders and presents with an extensive history of alcohol abuse. It is anticipated that if Frank were to be hospitalized or imprisoned, one of his most pressing concerns would be finding a way to secure medication to relieve the distress engendered by confinement. The problem with giving Frank medication is that distress is a direct consequence of lifestyle involvement, and to medicate his distress with an anxiolytic or antidepressant rather than using it to create a crisis and motivate change is countertherapeutic and a prime example of how the medical community enables lifestyle behavior. Whether a lifestyle revolves around drug abuse, crime, or marital infidelity, the use of psychotropic medication in individuals without serious Axis I psychopathology is contraindicated by the model described in this chapter.

11. Personal strengths.

The lifestyle model is at least as interested in uncovering a person's strengths as it is in exposing a person's weaknesses; Frank presents with a number of strengths that could be incorporated into a comprehensive program of change. First, Frank is free of any serious Axis I psychopathology aside from alcohol abuse, which is construed by proponents of the lifestyle approach as a lifestyle problem rather than an emotional or psychiatric disorder. The absence of significant psychopathology bodes well for any intervention that might be attempted with Frank in the sense that he is precluded from using emotional problems and difficulties to evade personal responsibility for his actions. Many individuals use real and imagined psychological difficulties to justify their continued involvement in a lifestyle pattern through mollification or entitlement, a practice that is sometimes reinforced by society even when the assertion is baseless (e.g., once an addict, always an addict). Freedom from psychopathology allows Frank to benefit from group sessions and to handle the confrontations that some of the more experienced members of the group are likely to direct his way. Good psychological adjustment signifies that Frank can participate fully in the lifestyle intervention process.

The case history discloses that Frank possesses above-average intellectual ability. This is another strength that can be used to promote change in a client like Frank, for like the absence of significant psychopathology it means that Frank can benefit from the full range of procedures offered by the lifestyle change model. The lifestyle change program, being largely educational in nature, is most effective when clients can comprehend the printed material that constitutes the bibliotherapy component of the program. Although the lifestyle approach can be simplified to give clients with low reading ability and significant intellectual deficits access to the information, in order to take full advantage of the program a person must possess at least average intellectual ability and an eighth grade reading level, both of which are well within Frank's grasp. Frank's above-average intelligence will also make it easier for him to appreciate the logic of the lifestyle approach. Rather than extolling moral principles (crime is wrong) lifestyle theorists have found it more effective, at least in North America, to emphasize practical matters (in most cases the benefits of crime do not outweigh the costs), provided the natural negative consequences of crime have taken effect. Once the enabling that has permitted Frank to engage in drug use and criminal behavior has been eliminated, he will be in a better position to learn from his mistakes.

A third personal strength that we might want to include in Frank's personalized program of change is his perceptiveness. Frank, as is mentioned throughout the case history, is proficient at identifying and capitalizing on a person's weaknesses for his own personal benefit or pleasure. It is argued that these skills can be turned around to serve more positive and pro-social objectives. First, Frank's perceptiveness implies that he has the capacity for empathy and perspective-taking. Those psychologists who would call Frank a psychopath (e.g., Hare, 1993) must explain why his sensitivity to other's feelings and perspective-taking skills are so strong given that lack of empathy is a defining characteristic of psychopathy. True, he presently uses these skills to manipulate rather than empathize, yet he is clearly not lacking in perceptiveness; rather, he just needs to learn how to channel these skills into positive pursuits. A helper who projects meaning and community as part of an evolving client-helper alliance could assist Frank in transforming his perceptiveness into a strength useful not only in understanding others but also in pointing to potential avenues of future employment in such areas as sales and marketing.

12. Addressing limits and boundaries.

During the first several sessions it is anticipated that Frank will attempt to subvert the therapeutic process by testing the boundaries and limits of the client-helper relationship and raising legitimate-sounding concerns about competence, accountability, and confidentiality that are nothing more than a manipulative ploy to avoid intimacy. He may well challenge the helper's credentials by asking to see a diploma or inquiring about qualifications, try the helper's patience by arriving late to sessions or missing sessions altogether, and strain the helper's resolve by introducing conflicts of confidentiality. This can best be handled by providing Frank with an overview of the limits and boundaries of therapy from the very first session and then reinforcing these limits and boundaries each time Frank violates them. Like a young child attempting to test a parent's love, Frank will defy the limits of the therapy relationship in order to discern whether the helper's offers of assistance are genuine. As the therapeutic relationship evolves, the testing of limits and boundaries will diminish rather than disappear. At this point Frank's testing efforts may become more covert and subtle as he seeks to establish an inappropriately close personal relationship with the helper designed to compromise the helper's objectivity. It is contingent upon whoever is conducting therapy with Frank that he or she remain steadfast in upholding the limits of therapy so that Frank can feel safe to explore the boundaries of his own belief systems in a psychologically protected environment.

13. Involving significant others and employing homework assignments.

The lifestyle approach to change is mindful of how people who have a significant impact on a client's life can serve as a source of reinforcement and limit-setting. In Frank's case this would include his wife and parole officer. Frank's wife Jennifer appears to be the only significant person he has left in his life. Perhaps this is because they have only been together a few years. The case history indicates that over the years Frank has burned the vast majority of his bridges with family and friends. It is no coincidence, then, that Jennifer appears naive and timid, for these are the characteristics that Frank probably looks for in a mate. Beyond her physical appearance what appeals most to Frank about Jennifer is her apparent willingness to accept his version of reality. This just said, Frank may have underestimated Jennifer, who shows signs of having caught on to some of his manipulations and is beginning to demand that she be treated with respect and consideration. There are at least two reasons why it may be helpful to include Jennifer in the intervention. First, she has been adversely affected by Frank's behavior yet continues to support him. The fact that she is now able to see through his charm makes her a potentially valuable source of information as to Frank's progress outside of therapy. Second, Jennifer is the one person who seems capable of exerting pressure on Frank to participate in sessions, which will be vital during the early phases of intervention when the therapeutic alliance is still in its infancy and Frank's motivation for change is low. If Frank's parole is not immediately revoked his parole officer can use the pending legal charges as leverage to keep him from dropping out of therapy. While it is true that people cannot be forced to change, it is sometimes necessary to bring external pressure to bear on a person with a drug or crime problem for him or her to remain active in therapy prior to development of a therapeutic relationship.

Homework assignments assume a prominent position in the lifestyle approach to change, for they allow application of information discussed in therapy to real-life situations and events. With respect to the problem-solving component of Frank's change program, the helper could instruct Frank to identify a problem during the session and outline a solution to the problem with the problem-solving technique during the week. The outcome of the homework assignment could then be discussed at the next regularly scheduled session. The assertiveness component of Frank's change plan is designed to build Frank's confidence in his ability to handle situations that characteristically trigger anger. Lessons learned in interaction with the helper and other group members can be reinforced and extended to real-life situations by having Frank practice his assertiveness skills in real-life situations, first with a safe person like his wife and later with a stranger such as a waiter at a restaurant where he is instructed to send back an undercooked steak. In helping Frank find new meaning in life it may be discovered that cognitive indolence, as represented by Frank's proclivity for conspiratorial thinking, is a major feature of his self- and world-views. The cognitive restructuring he receives in therapy can be reinforced with a homework assignment where he is instructed to critically evaluate a half dozen television commercials during the week and in the next session discuss the methods the sponsors used to persuade viewers to purchase their product. Finally, the social interest that Frank has been cultivating in an effort to achieve community could be reinforced with a homework assignment that requires him to implement one of the three ways he had previously identified to help out his wife.

14. Termination and relapse prevention.

After 6 to 24 months of weekly individual and/or group sessions it is anticipated that the subject of therapy termination will need to be broached. Rather than a sudden discontinuation of sessions it makes more sense to schedule three to five booster sessions at 3 to 4 week intervals to provide Frank with the support and guidance he needs to resist the temptation of a drug or criminal lifestyle. It may not be a bad idea to include Frank's wife Jennifer in a number of these booster sessions, for it is anticipated that she will become Frank's primary source of social support once therapy ends. If agreeable to both parties I might be inclined to see Frank and Jennifer together in couples therapy for several months prior to termination and for all or most of the booster sessions. Social support remains the single best predictor of outcome in clients releasing from substance abuse programming (Booth, Russell, Soucek, & Laughlin, 1992; Higgins, Budney, Bickel, & Badger, 1994) and it is a prime consideration when planning the termination of a therapeutic relationship with a substance abusing or crime-involved client.

Relapse prevention is often stressed several months prior to the cessation of lifestyle intervention and normally includes a relapse prevention plan. The relapse prevention plan employed in lifestyle therapy is modeled after the change plans that are used throughout the lifestyle change process (Walters, 1998b). Lifestyle theory rejects the medical model concept of treatment and with it the notion of a treatment plan imposed by an outside expert. A change plan, by comparison, is constructed by the client with assistance from the helper whose job it is to make sure the information is as specific and behavioral as possible. The change plan covers three areas: involvements (the activities a person engages in and the people with whom he or she associates), commitments (the goals and values a person pursues), and identifications (how a person perceives himself or herself), each of which are divided into time frames (past, present, and future) to yield nine boxes. By the time he nears termination Frank might respond to the involvement section of the change plan as follows: past involvements—drinking in bars and conducting phony business deals; present involvements—spending time with my wife and looking for legitimate employment; future involvements—raising and providing for my family. The change plan is completed periodically, even after formal therapy ends, and reinforces the perspective that change is a never-ending process.

15. Mechanisms for change.

The principal mechanism for change according to lifestyle theory is the human organism's natural capacity for change. Humans, like all living organisms, are open systems in the sense that they freely exchange energy with the environment. Such energy exchange gives rise to the nonlinear dynamical systems concept of self-organization, which is the capacity of dynamic systems to generate new forms through ongoing interaction with the environment (Walters, 1999). Change, then, is a natural consequence of the human organism's daily interactions with the environment. However, for every thesis there is an antithesis and for every force a counterforce. The opposing force to change is the desire for continuation or pattern continuity (Walters, 2002b), which is why most people fear change. Lifestyle theory recommends using events in a person's life to devise life lessons and crises capable of overriding a person's natural fear of change. Frank's fear of change, in fact, is what keeps him locked into a drug and criminal lifestyle. Using the natural negative consequences of Frank's lifestyle to alter the balance between continuity and change is a prime example of how resistance to change can be overcome in someone dependent on a lifestyle to manage the problems of everyday living.

The human organism is designed for change, but it does not follow that all change is in the best interests of the organism. Change as a means of strengthening adaptability, the principal goal of lifestyle intervention, requires direction and guidance, specifically, the guidance of a trained helper who through the formation of a therapeutic alliance and supporting-shaman effect steers the client toward the four key elements of change: responsibility, confidence, meaning, and community. The four key elements foster change by encouraging self-reliance and interdependence rather than lifestyle servitude and social isolation. Adaptive change may be directed by an interpersonal process, yet a trained helper is not always required. If Frank's wife was more assertive or if he had a better relationship with his brother either one could serve as the source of interpersonal influence for a personal program of adaptive change; after all, most people exit a drug or criminal lifestyle without professional help (Walters, 1998a, 2000d). As it turns out, the best option for change in Frank's case is a trained helper, combined with reduced enabling from Frank's wife and pressure from his parole officer to shift the balance of power toward change and away from continuity.

The principal mechanism of change is the natural change process, which commonly requires stimulation and guidance from an interpersonal relationship that encourages responsibility, confidence, meaning, and community. Specific therapeutic techniques are secondary to the natural change process and helping relationship but they can nevertheless be instrumental in facilitating change. No two people are exactly alike and so each intervention calls for a unique set of therapeutic tools and strategies. In Frank's case the techniques that are most likely to prove beneficial are those that teach him better decision-making skills (problem-solving training), furnish him with alternative coping strategies (stress and anger management), challenge prominent thinking styles like mollification, cutoff, power orientation, and cognitive indolence (rational restructuring), and help him develop concern for the welfare of others (social interest). Techniques that are effective with Frank may be useless or redundant with someone else. Consequently, lifestyle interventions are never carbon copies of one another. This individualized approach contrasts sharply with the typical inpatient treatment program for substance abuse where Frank would have been assigned a standard treatment protocol under the assumption that he suffered from the disease of alcoholism which responds uniformly to the same set of procedures.

CONCLUSION

After describing the lifestyle approach to change, the model was applied to Frank, the case study upon which this book is based. Given that Frank displays significant problems with both alcohol and crime, and since research indicates that drugs and crime are often reciprocally rather than unilaterally related, the lifestyle approach, in which Frank's drinking and antisocial behavior can be addressed contemporaneously, was seen as a cost-effective alternative to traditional therapies and interventions. As the present discussion bears out, an array of specific techniques are utilized by professionals employing the lifestyle model of change, but these techniques are secondary to the therapeutic alliance that facilitates the natural process believed to exist in all people and which is most reliably accessed through the four key elements of responsibility, confidence, meaning, and community. The ultimate goal of lifestyle intervention is to help the individual alter his or her reality by modifying core belief systems through an interpersonal process in which the four key elements of change serve as beacons for self-organization.

REFERENCES

Adler, A. (1973). *Superiority and social interest: A collection of later writings* (H. L. Ansbacher & R. R. Ansbacher, Eds.). New York: Viking Press.

Beck, A. T., Wright, F. D., Newman, C. F., & Liese, B. S. (1993). *Cognitive therapy of substance abuse*. New York: Guilford.

Booth, B. M., Russell, D. W., Soucek, S., & Laughlin, P. R. (1992). Social support and outcome of alcoholism treatment: An exploratory analysis. *American Journal of Drug and Alcohol Abuse, 18*, 87–101.

Cleckley, H. (1976). *The mask of sanity* (5th ed.). St. Louis, MO: Mosby. (Original work published 1941)

Ellis, A., & Dryden, W. (1997). *The practice of rational emotive therapy* (2nd ed.). New York: Springer.

Hare, R. D. (1993). *Without conscience: The disturbing world of the psychopaths among us*. New York: Pocket Books.

Higgins, S. T., Budney, A. J., Bickel, W. K., & Badger, G. J. (1994). Participation of significant others in outpatient behavioral treatment predicts greater cocaine abstinence. *American Journal of Drug and Alcohol Abuse, 20*, 47–56.

Lewis, M., & Brooks-Gunn, J. (1979). *Social cognition and the acquisition of the self*. New York: Plenum.

Marlatt, G. A., Larimer, M. E., Baer, J. S., & Quigley, L. A. (1993). Harm reduction for alcohol problems: Moving beyond the controlled drinking controversy. *Behavior Therapy, 24*, 461–504.

Miller, W. R. (1985). Motivation for treatment: A review with special emphasis on alcoholism. *Psychological Bulletin, 98*, 84–107.

Piaget, J. (1952). *The origins of intelligence in children*. New York: International Universities Press.

Shover, N. (1996). *Great pretenders: Pursuits and careers of persistent thieves*. Oxford, UK: Westview.

Walters, G. D. (1994). Discriminating between high and low volume substance abusers by means of the Drug Lifestyle Screening Interview. *American Journal of Drug and Alcohol Abuse, 20,* 19–33.

Walters, G. D. (1995). The Psychological Inventory of Criminal Thinking Styles: Part I. Reliability and preliminary validity. *Criminal Justice and Behavior, 22,* 307–325.

Walters, G. D. (1998a). *Changing lives of drugs and crime: Intervening with substance-abusing offenders.* Chichester, UK: Wiley.

Walters, G. D. (1998b). Planning for change: An alternative to treatment planning with sexual offenders. *Journal of Sex and Marital Therapy, 24,* 217–229.

Walters, G. D. (1999). Crime and chaos: Applying nonlinear dynamical principles to problems in criminology. *International Journal of Offender Therapy and Comparative Criminology, 43,* 134–153.

Walters, G. D. (2000a). Behavioral self-control training for problem drinkers: A meta-analysis of randomized control studies. *Behavior Therapy, 31,* 135–149.

Walters, G. D. (2000b). *Beyond behavior: Construction of an overarching psychological theory of lifestyles.* Westport, CT: Praeger.

Walters, G. D. (2000c). *The self-altering process: Exploring the dynamic nature of lifestyle development and change.* Westport, CT: Praeger.

Walters, G. D. (2000d). Spontaneous remission from alcohol, tobacco, and other drug abuse: Seeking quantitative answers to qualitative questions. *American Journal of Drug and Alcohol Abuse, 26,* 443–460.

Walters, G. D. (2001). The shaman effect in counseling clients with alcohol problems. *Alcoholism Treatment Quarterly, 19*(3), 31–43.

Walters, G. D. (2002b). Maintaining motivation for change using resources available in an offender's natural environment. In M. McMurran (Ed.), *Motivating offenders to change: A guide to enhancing engagement in therapy* (pp. 121–135). Chichester, England: Wiley.

Walters, G. D., White, T. W., & Denney, D. (1991). The Lifestyle Criminality Screening Form: Preliminary data. *Criminal Justice and Behavior, 18,* 406–418.

Walters, G. D., & Willoughby, F. W. (2000). The Psychological Inventory of Drug-Based Thinking Styles (PIDTS): Preliminary data. *Alcoholism Treatment Quarterly, 18*(2), 51–66.

Yochelson, S., Samenow, S. E. (1976). *The criminal personality: Vol. 1. A profile for change.* New York: Aronson.

CHAPTER 7

The Cognitive Behavioral Treatment Approach

Arthur Freeman and Brian Eig

I. Treatment Model

Individuals with personality disorders, regardless of the type, test the patience and frustration tolerance of many of those who come into contact with them. They especially test the patience and skills of therapists trying to treat them. Although a commonly held belief among therapists is that individuals with Antisocial Personality Disorder (ASPD) do not and cannot benefit from psychotherapy, this chapter offers a suggestion that Cognitive-Behavioral Therapy (CBT) can provide a strategic and collaborative way of reaching this difficult to treat population.

Although psychological literature is filled with an abundance of research which clarifies the definition, assessment, and description of the various typologies of ASPD, the literature on treating such challenging behavior is scarce at best. However, the cost to society of not developing an effective treatment protocol for people with antisocial traits or full-blown personality disorders is astronomical.

CBT provides a structured approach that focuses on the composite of related beliefs and behaviors often manifested by persons with personality disorders (Beck, Freeman, Davis, and Associates, 2004, p. 163). "Cognitive therapy is based on a straightforward, commonsense model of the relationships among cognition, emotion, and behavior in human functioning in general and in psychopathology in particular" (Freeman, Pretzer, Fleming, & Simon, 1990, p. 4).

In general, three main areas of cognition become the targets of intervention. These include: (1) Automatic Thoughts, (2) Core Beliefs (Schemas), and (3) Cognitive Distortions. Cognitive theory holds that thoughts, feelings, and behaviors are reciprocal and interdependent. In other words, thoughts impact emotions, and emotions influence thoughts and behaviors. Likewise, "behaviors can influence the evaluation of a situation by modifying the situation itself or by eliciting responses from others" (Freeman et al., 2004, p. 6).

When using CBT to treat personality disorders, a greater emphasis is placed on changing the patient's core beliefs, rather than his/her dysfunctional thoughts (Roy & Tyrer, 2001). Because Frank's maladaptive beliefs appear stable and consistent across different settings, his schema are expected to manifest similarly in the therapeutic relationship. The therapeutic relationship can be used as a "relationship laboratory" as Frank is helped to learn new and more adaptive ways of relating to others (Roy & Tyrer,). Thus, the first challenge facing the therapist working with the patient with an ASPD is in establishing and maintaining a stable, therapeutic alliance.

The worldview of an individual with ASPD is quite different from that of the non-ASPD population. According to Beck and associates (2004, p. 167) the view of the world from an antisocial perspective is a "personal" rather than "interpersonal" view. People such as Frank have great difficulty taking on the perspective of another. They tend to think in a linear, goal-directed, and concrete way, anticipating the reactions of others only after responding to their own needs and desires (Beck et al., p. 167).

Cognitive theorists stress that it is usually more productive to identify and modify core problems when treating individuals with personality disorders (Freeman & Jackson, 1998, p. 320). "The schemata of individuals with a personality disorder are so vivid and obvious that they may appear to be a caricature of what one would expect in 'normal' individuals" (Freeman & Jackson, p. 322.). The feelings and behaviors of antisocial individuals can be conceptualized as functioning within certain schema which produce consistently biased judgments and a concomitant tendency to make cognitive errors in a variety of situations (Freeman & Jackson, p. 322).

> Often, the hallmark of a personality disorder is "other blaming". The personality disordered patient will often see the difficulties that they encounter in dealing with other people or coping with life tasks as externally generated and independent of their behavior. Much of what they experience is, in their view, "done to them" or generally coming from the ill-will or negative actions of those around them. This 'other blaming' position often places them in conflict with peers, and often puts them in conflict with larger agencies and institutions (Freeman & Jackson, 1998, p. 322).

According to Young (1994) the origins of a personality disorder can be traced back to the development of early maladaptive schemas. These schemas are defined as "broad, pervasive themes regarding oneself and one's relationship with others, developed during childhood and elaborated throughout one's lifetime and dysfunctional to a significant degree" (Young, p. 209). "In some cases the behavior that is now part of the Axis II disorder has been functional in life." (Freeman & Jackson, 1998, p. 322).

Young (1994) further suggests that schemas of entitlement/grandiosity and insufficient self-control/self-discipline lead to deficiencies in the ability to maintain internal limits, assume responsibility to others, and/or orient the individual to long-term goals.

A specific type of CBT, Schema Focused Therapy, may be useful when working with Frank. Schema Focused Therapy can be conceptualized as having two distinct phases. In the first phase, called the "Assessment" phase, the therapist and patient focus on the identification and activation of particular schemas (Young, 2003, p. 209). This is followed by the "Change" phase, where the therapist attempts to modify the relevant schemas by altering the distorted view of the self and others.

During the assessment phase of treatment the therapist focuses on two critical tasks. The first task, schema identification, requires that the therapist and patient identify the schemas that are relevant to the ASPD. In elaborating the schema, the therapist should identify how the schema is maintained, avoided, and/or compensated for, which may lead to productive avenues of exploration.

The second task is "Schema Activation," where the therapist seeks to trigger affect associated with the identified schema. Here the patient may be asked to use imagery to elicit childhood scenes of interactions with various significant people in his life.

> "In essence, the role of the therapist is to help the patient tolerate low levels of schema-related affect and then gradually intensify the experience until the patient is able to tolerate the full imagery exercise without retreating from the image (Yong, 2003, p. 210)."

Although CBT with personality-disordered patients tends to focus on the patients' core belief, there is still attention given to automatic thoughts inasmuch as the automatic thoughts stem from and reflect schemas related to pragmatic strategies for self-advancement or self-preservation. A common underlying goal for antisocial individuals is to limit and/or avoid the real or perceived sense of being controlled by others (Beck et al., 2004).

Further, the antisocial individual typically maintains a number of beliefs that serve to guide his/her behavior. These frequently include, but are not limited to, the following beliefs (or combinations and derivatives):

- **Justification**—"Wanting something (or wanting to avoid something) justifies my actions."
- **Thinking is believing**—"My thoughts and feelings are completely accurate, simply because they occur to me."
- **Personal infallibility**—"I always make good choices."
- **Feelings make facts**—"I know I am right because I feel right about what I do."
- **Impotence of others**—"The views of others are irrelevant to my decisions, unless they can directly control my immediate consequences."
- **Low-impact consequences**—"If there are undesirable consequences they will not matter to me."
- **Narcissism**—"I am more special than all others."
- **Lack of empathy**—"I do not have to worry about others."
- **Lack of societal focus**—"Rules are for fools."
- **Lack of (or flawed) information**—"There are many places in the world where my behavior is acceptable.

(Adapted from Beck et al., 2004)

It would be naïve for the therapist to assume that the patient with ASPD is coming to therapy with the intent of changing. Often they are sent for therapy as an alternative to incarceration. Further, the antisocial behavior has likely been reinforced by others or by society in rewarding the individual for their antisocial actions. For example, a patient jailed for selling drugs was referred for therapy as a condition of his probation. He parked in the clinic parking lot next to the therapist's car. The patient had a new, high-end SUV and the therapist was driving a 10-year-old import. The patient started the session by commenting, "Nice wheels, doc." Another issue for consideration is that for many individuals with personality disorders, the pervasive nature of the disorder has led to limited or absent skill repertoire. The major skill deficit for the ASPD is empathy. They have learned limited perspective taking. Finally, a problem exists within the DSM-IV-TR nosology (American Psychiatric Association, 2000). The diagnosis of ASPD requires the following, " . . . .a pervasive pattern of disregard for and violation of the rights of others since the age of 15 years . . . " (p. 706). Further, " . . . the individual must be at least 18 years (Criterion B) and must have had a history of some symptoms of Conduct Disorder before age 15 years (Criterion C)" (p. 702).

The report, however, of early conduct-disordered behavior, absent "official" legal, school, or clinical reports, is most frequently from an individual where " . . . deceit and manipulation are central features of the Antisocial Personality Disorder . . . ." (p. 702). The patient may deny early conduct-disordered behavior or embellish an extensive history if they believe that it is to their advantage to manipulate the data.

II. Clinical skills most essential to successful therapy

Before launching into treatment with individuals who present intense characterological difficulties, a therapist should consider his or her readiness as well as willingness to take on such a challenge. The therapist must have the ability to tolerate the potentiality of highly negative emotions. Likewise, the therapist must be able to monitor his/her own automatic and often negative emotional responses to the patient (Beck et al., 2004, p. 169). "The therapist must be able to control his/her responses to the patient's often angry, demeaning, or hostile verbalizations or behavior and not become pejorative or inflexible in response" (p. 170). A full understanding of personality disorders, especially of the ASPD patient, is particularly necessary to be able to work effectively with a case such as Frank. "The idea that a patient with ASPD is like all other patients, just more difficult, is a massive under-evaluation" (Beck et al., p. 169). Therapists should be aware of the long-term, chronic, and pervasive nature of personality disorders, while understanding that maladaptive schemas of the personality-disordered patient are not easily changed. This knowledge can help a therapist deal with the frustrations that often follow what may otherwise be considered treatment failures.

It also takes a unique, therapeutic style to work with personality-disordered patients, one that fits well with their way of viewing the world. It takes a great deal of experience and skill to work effectively with personality-disordered patients. The more the therapist does it the better they get at doing it. However, for even the master therapist, supervision or consultation is s a crucial aspect necessary to keep the clinician supported, sharp, focused, and on target.

"The therapist treating the patient with APD must be trained to work with the problems of anger, dissociation, dishonesty, and relationship difficulty, often within the context of an unstable working alliance" (Beck et al., 2004, p. 170). He or she must also have patience, perseverance, and the ability not to take the patient's reactions personally. While continuing to maintain hope for the patient, the therapist must resist the temptation to be drawn into the patient's own sense of impatience, frustration, futility, and drama.

Another important skill for a therapist to have is good timing. Even the best interventions that are poorly timed may become counterproductive in therapy (Freeman & Jackson, 1998, p. 334). Furthermore, the therapist must be able to maintain a high level of focus and attention. Individuals with ASPD often present with a friendly, even charming, demeanor that can disarm the naïve therapist and interfere with his/her objectivity. The patient may gloss over important topics with vague or incomplete answers and a dismissive smile. They may make the therapist feel silly about asking certain questions, as if they were so obvious or unimportant that a "good therapist" should know better. ("Are you kidding asking me that?") On the other hand, ASPD patients may become threatening or frightening, tempting clinicians to gloss over important questions, skip details, and shorten interviews ("Hey! Watch it! That's none of your damn business.") (Reid, 2001).

A final conceptual issue is helping the patient develop the motivation for change. In what way is it to the patient's advantage to do things differently? Unless change is viewed as valuable for the patient, little will be done in the direction of altering behavior.

Freeman, Saxon-Hunt, and Yacono (2004) identify a number of factors that must be taken into account in the treatment. These are:

1. The therapist must have an extensive understanding of the nature of personality disorders.
2. The patient must be helped to understand the life impact and the implications of having an antisocial personality disorder.
3. The therapist must be aware of the likely resistance to change.
4. The therapist and the patient must have the requisite skills to cope with a personality disorder.
5. Both patient and therapist must have the motivation to manage the ongoing challenges in the treatment of a personality disorder.
6. The therapist must be able to deal with frustration stemming from the therapy.
7. Both therapist and patient must work on developing a support network for the "difficult days" ahead.
8. The therapist must maintain the structure necessary and inherent in CBT.
9. Both therapist and patient must be able to maintain the therapeutic collaboration through the "bad days."
10. The therapist must help the patient develop an optimistic view of the future.

11. Early and often, the therapist must set out realistic, observable, and measurable goals for therapy.
12. The patient needs to be helped to develop the motivation and skills to control anger and impulsive behavior.
13. The patient needs to be helped to develop the motivation and skills necessary for taking a problem-solving approach to situations.
14. The therapist and patient must develop the "vision" to see problems on the horizon and be able to head them off in an adaptive manner.
15. The patient needs to be able to effectively self-monitor.
16. The patient needs to be able to take the perspective of others and to monitor their reactions.
17. The therapist must be able to motivate the patient to use homework as a major therapeutic tool.
18. The patient will need to develop skills for dealing with the anxiety that will likely be raised in the course of the therapy.
19. The patient and the therapist must agree on the boundaries that will be maintained in the therapy.
20. Both therapist and patient must be willing to seek help, as needed.

Therapeutic Questions
1. What are the therapeutic goals for this patient?

Well-defined goals and objectives are the foundation of good therapy. As such, when working with Frank, it would be imperative to establish clear and measurable goals. Identifying long-term goals, with proximal sub-goals and objectives, serves to maintain a clear direction and focus for treatment. "It is important to remember that the patient's goals and not those of others (including the therapist), are the initial focus of treatment" (Freeman & Jackson, 1998, p. 321).

The therapeutic relationship will be a microcosm of the patients' responses to others in their environment. When working with Frank, we would want to begin building rapport, while orienting him to the structure of cognitive-behavioral therapy, the expected outcomes and time course, as well as the procedures and strategies that will be used.

As an initial strategy for the onset of therapy, it would be beneficial, especially considering that Frank is being court-mandated into therapy, to work on an immediate problem, thereby striving to create the mindset for Frank that therapy could have value after all, and that it may be worthwhile continuing to work in therapy.

Marlowe and Sugarman (1997) address the importance of setting dual goals for individuals with antisocial personalities. They recommend that improved problem-solving ability should be the focus of short-term goals, with increased motivation for change being the goals for the long-term.

Based on the extreme difficulties that Frank's impulsive behavior creates for himself, another goal would be to improve his self-control. Having socially acceptable self-control would allow Frank to accomplish useful work and preserve what has been a long history of tenuous social bonds (Strayhorn, 2002b). The overarching goal for Frank would therefore be to give him a more pro-social way of interacting with others (Robinson, 2003, p. 67).

2. What further information and tools are needed to structure treatment?

Structured therapy sessions are an essential component of CBT. In order to make the most efficient use of time the therapy session should follow a relatively standard format. We would recommend developing an agenda for each session. This would allow both the therapist and the patient to decide what will be worked on during that session. Afterwards, the focus may switch to the patient's current status and significant events of the week, feedback regarding last session, main agenda items, developing new homework, and finally eliciting feedback about the current session (Freeman, Pretzer, Fleming, & Simon, 1990). Based upon his focus and practice of collaboration with patients, Beck referred to the therapeutic process as "collaborative empiricism" (Beck, Rush, Shaw, & Emery, 1979). In the spirit of collaborative empiricism, we would try to work with Frank as a "team," systematically exploring and testing his thoughts and beliefs.

Another important aspect of CBT is the emphasis placed on outcome measurement. The question arises as to how progress will be measured with Frank? Three tools are recommended: (1) Psychopathic Checklist—Revised (PCL—R), (2) Schema Conceptualization Form, and (3) The Freeman Diagnostic Profiling System.

The PCL—R is a commonly used, 20 item, instrument for measuring antisocial (referred to here as psychopathic) behaviors as well as affective and interpersonal indicators. Since, by definition, antisocial individuals have a tendency to easily and frequently lie, the PCL—R incorporates collateral information, resulting in highly reliable scores (Brinkley, Newman, Widiger, & Lynam, 2004). Brinkley and associates also refer to the PCL—R as the "gold standard" measure of antisocial personality.

The Schema Conceptualization Form (as in Young, 2002) is an instrument which guides the therapist through the complicated process of viewing the patient's problems in "schema terms," helping to form an effective treatment plan and clear direction for therapy.

The Freeman Diagnostic Profiling System uses the diagnostic criteria of DSM-IV-TR as a technique for assessment and for structuring treatment (Freeman & Jackson, 1998)

Using these three instruments, we would predictably obtain a quantifiable profile of Frank which would yield measurable baseline information regarding his behaviors (impulsivity), affective concerns (shallowness of emotions), interpersonal issues (superficiality), as well as diagnostic criteria and treatment plan goals/objectives. By using these scores as a baseline measure, Frank could be re-assessed at a later point in therapy to determine if and to what extent changes and progress have been achieved.

3. What is your conceptualization of this patient's personality, behavior, affective state, and cognitions?

"The case formulation is the therapist's compass; it guides the treatment" (Persons, 1989, p. 37). The most important function of the conceptualization is to provide the basis for the treatment plan, which follows directly from the hypothesis about the nature of the underlying deficit producing the patient's problems. According to Persons, psychological problems can be conceptualized as occurring at two levels: the overt difficulties and the underlying psychological mechanisms (p. 1). Overt difficulties represent the "real life" problems that patients such as Frank experience, and include difficulty getting along with others, inability to maintain employment, impulsivity, or poor affective modulation. Underlying psychological mechanisms, on the other hand, are the psychological deficits that underlie and cause the overt difficulties (p. 1).

> The case formulation has six parts: (1) the problem list, (2) the proposed underlying mechanism, (3) an account of the way in which the proposed mechanism produces the problems on the problem list, (4) precipitants of current problems, (5) origins of the mechanism in the patient's early life, and, (6) predicted obstacles to treatment based on the formulation (Persons, 1989, p. 48).

Based on interviews with significant people in Frank's life, the follow problem list could be developed:

1. Poor self-control
2. Thrill-seeking behavior (with little regard for the safety of self and others)

3. Superficial and exploitive relationships
4. Irresponsible behavior
5. Difficulty with authority
6. Other blaming.

Frank's problem meets the DSM-IV-TR diagnostic criteria for Antisocial Personality Disorder,

The underlying mechanism which seems to cause Frank's difficulties can be explained by identifying his relevant schemas. What schemas would account for Frank's behavior? Is there a common theme? What core beliefs would someone hold who acts in the way Frank does? A possible hypothesis could be a schema such as, "Everything should revolve around my happiness and pleasure" and "Wanting something justifies my actions."

With these schemas in mind, Frank's behaviors make sense. Rules, for people such as Frank, are an annoyance and obstacles to be overcome. If Frank's core belief is that his happiness supercedes anyone else's needs, his behavior, regardless of whether it appears "right or wrong," is more easily understood. Furthermore, if Frank believes that "rules are for fools," and that rules interfere with his pursuit of happiness, what would be the justification for following those rules? As such, Frank has had little need for, nor has he ever developed, very good self-control (problem #1). Likewise, Frank has a high need for stimulation. On the surface, this doesn't sound like a dangerous thing; however, when we add the schematic component, we can see that Frank's stimulation or thrill-seeking comes at the expense of his and others' safety (problem #2). His schema also clearly frames his problem of superficial and exploitative relationships (problem #3) as well as his irresponsible behavior (problem #4). Furthermore, someone who is seen as an authority figure is, in Frank's mind, someone who would want to stop the good times, further explaining why he and authority do not mix (problem #5). Similarly, because Frank has difficulty taking the perspective of another, when problems arise, they aren't seen as his problems. Frank just wants to have fun and be happy! It's the rest of the world that is screwed up (problem #6).

In seeking to identify the origin of Frank's core beliefs, we would look to Frank's family origin. According to Strayhorn (2002b), a kind yet firm parent seems to foster self-control in the child. In contrast, Frank's upbringing by an abusive and sadistic father is far from a good role model of self-control. Moreover, as observed in many antisocial youth, it is hypothesized that the failure to delay gratification arises from an absence of trustworthy relationships, which makes it rational to delay gratification rather than to "get what you can now," because you can't count on anything or anybody in the future. Therefore we can predict, although one can never say for sure whether antisocial traits are developed from nurture or nature, that Frank learned how to deal with an abusive and inconsistent parent by developing schemas regarding how to get his needs met. Frank may hold the schema, "I got to get what I can because I can't rely on anyone."

4. What potential pitfalls would you envision in this therapy? What would the difficulties be and what would you envision to be the sources of the difficulties?

Several patient characteristics must be assumed in order for Frank to benefit from CBT. These include:

- Rready access to thoughts and feelings
- Having identifiable life problems to focus on
- The ability and willingness to do homework assignments
- Engagement in a collaborative relationship with the therapist
- Cognitions that are flexible enough to be modified.

It is questionable whether Frank would meet these conditions. To the extent that he would not, Young (2002) suggests that therapy would often fail without significant schematic alterations. It is also important to keep in mind that people with ASPD represent an extremely diverse, heterogeneous population. Therefore, no single treatment strategy can be recommended for any single disorder (Oldham, 1994). In other words, there is no single treatment that would work with all antisocial individuals. Modifications to therapy in order to fit the needs of the individual will always have to be made.

Another anticipated obstacle pertains to the fact that Frank sees his problems as other people's inability to accept him or the desire of others to limit his freedom (Beck et al., 2004, p. 169). Therefore, we would have to identify even the smallest ambivalence Frank may entertain in order to find a foothold for increasing his motivation for treatment.

As difficult as it might be, we would have to be "morally neutral" when working with Frank. We would also be careful not to do anything that could be misconstrued as approval for his antisocial acts, or risk being interpreted by Frank as a partner in crime or of being in "collusion" (Robinson, 2003, p. 60). Though easier said than done, this can be accomplished by focusing strictly on Frank's behaviors rather than on Frank the person.

Difficulties will likely begin when Frank's attempts at manipulation are resisted, or his requests/demands are not fulfilled (Robinson, 2003, p. 60). It would not be surprising for Frank to then become verbally hostile, critical, derogatory, intimidating, or possibly even violent toward the therapist.

If rapport is lost or difficult to initiate, it may be obtained by appealing to Frank's sense of grandiosity. Given Frank's "style" of being at the center of attention, he may respond to an air of indifference on our part. One of the most important treatment considerations in working with personality disordered individuals is to be aware that when the therapy approaches the active and compelling schema we will invoke anxiety (Freeman & Jackson, 1998). This anxiety will likely trigger a negative schematic mode for Frank, resulting in a surge of negative affect.

5. To what level of coping, adaptation, or function would you see this patient reaching as an immediate result of therapy? What result would be long-term subsequent to the ending of therapy? Prognosis for adaptive change?

How much and what type of adaptive change is likely with Frank will be a key issue in our selecting goals and interventions. Beck and associates (2004) conceptualize cognitive therapy as improving moral and social behavior through the enhancement of cognitive functioning. "Cognitive therapy is designed to help a patient with ASPD make a transition from thinking in mostly concrete, immediate terms considering a broader spectrum of interpersonal perspectives, alternative beliefs, and possible actions" (p. 169).

Freeman and Jackson (1998) identified four types of schematic change, ranging from the most drastic change (schematic restructuring) to a more surface level change (schematic camouflage). Schematic restructuring refers to the breaking down and rebuilding of a completely new personality structure. It may be overly ambitious if not foolhardy to strive for this type of restructuring when working with someone such as Frank. An example of schematic restructuring is to have Frank become a fully trusting and prosocial individual. Anyone who expects to come out of therapy as a totally different person will inevitably be disappointed. To the list we would add schematic construction, that is, building new schema from the ground up.

The next level of schematic change involves smaller changes in the way that Frank views his world. An example would be to have Frank modify the idea that "people cannot be trusted" to "in many cases people cannot be totally trusted." Although this type of change is more realistic, the fact remains that Frank's belief system is highly inflexible, long-standing, and well-imbedded. It is unlikely that therapy will result in this type of change with Frank.

Schematic reinterpretation would involve helping Frank reinterpret his schema in more functional ways. This may be a more realistic goal for Frank. Essentially, Frank may learn to use his schema in ways that help rather than hurt himself and others. Finally, the most likely outcome of therapy would be what is considered schematic camouflage, that is, acting differently, whether of nor he believes in what he is doing. Frank can be helped to act in a more empathic manner. He could possibly maintain this were there no external stressors that cause him to slip back. Although this is a more superficial and surface level of change, it would allow Frank to adapt and function in his environment in more pro-social ways. Schematic camouflage involves the patient testing new ways of behaving, with or without full understanding of the principle differences, but still resulting in more acceptable interpersonal interactions.

According to Ochman (1999), patients such as Frank may never develop empathy, but they may learn a safer, more responsible form of social behavior. In operational terms, the changes we would hope to see may include his curbing of impulses in order to comply with societal rules, engaging in less aggressive styles of conflict resolution, and being able to use techniques to calm himself rather than having an emotional outburst. Strayhorn (2002a) identifies other behavioral changes, such as choosing to tell the truth even though lying would feel more familiar and comfortable, showing up for appointments he would rather skip, and complying with often tedious day-to-day responsibilities. While we agree with Strayhorn, we would not want to push our luck this far with Frank.

6. What would be your timeline (duration) for therapy? What would be the frequency and duration of sessions?

"It is crucial for therapists to convey to patients that, although the personality disorder is a chronic condition, it can be highly treatable" (Beck et al., 2004, p. 171). In addition, it may be helpful for Frank to know that his level of motivation for change will be a contributing factor related to his therapeutic success.

For us to work effectively with Frank, we would need to be flexible in our therapeutic techniques, as well as in the duration and frequency of sessions. By their very nature, personality disorders will take more time to treat than other types of disorders. Freeman and Jackson (1998) suggest that a reasonable time-frame for therapy of personality disorders could be anywhere from 12 to 20 months. This is not "cure" time, but rather "adaptation" time.

Perry, Banon, and Ianni (1999) conducted a meta-analysis on the duration of treatment for people with personality disorders. Although results were highly variable, the authors identified a median period of treatment to be approximately 40 sessions over 28 weeks. Unfortunately, people with ASPD have a very high dropout rate. Researchers have predicted that treatment duration of less than 16 weeks will result in dropout rates of 8.2%. However, the longer treatment continues, logically, the higher dropout rates become. Perry and associates identified a 29.3% dropout rate when treatment continued past 16 weeks.

Further meta-analysis suggested that 92 treatment sessions or 1.3 years of treatment would yield recovery from personality disorder according to the full criteria in 50% of mixed personality disorder subjects (Perry et al., 1999). By comparison, the authors suggest that without treatment it would take 10.5 years to yield recovery in 50% of individuals.

Psychotherapy is associated with a sevenfold faster rate of recovery compared to the naturalistic studies (Perry et al., 1999). Without treatment, estimated recovery rates are about 3.7% per year, and with active treatment the rates increase to 25.8% per year (Perry et al.). Further estimates suggest that 25% of patients with personality disorder would recover by about 0.4 years, 50% by 1.3 years or 92 sessions, and 75% by 2.2 years or about 216 sessions (Perry et al.).

So how long would Frank be expected to remain in treatment? Only a broad range can be offered. Based on one session per week, treatment duration would be expected to take at least 12 months. However, if Frank continued in therapy until all his goals were achieved, he might be in treatment for twice that amount of time. Unfortunately, many people such as Frank do not complete therapy.

7. Are there specific or special techniques that you would implement in the therapy? What would they be?

As mentioned previously, a hallmark of CBT is the active and collaborative relationship between the patient and therapist. We would advocate an approach in which Frank is trained to develop skills that promote self-arguments to combat his manifest cognitive distortions.

Each session of CBT with Frank would commence with the setting of a collaborative agenda. At the beginning of the therapy, we would explain to Frank the importance of utilizing his valuable time in the most advantageous and efficient manner. Thus, we would strive for a therapeutic partnership right from the start of therapy. We could begin the process of agenda-setting by listing those areas that will be covered during the initial session, including: (a) identification of the concerns from Frank's point of view, (b) Frank's hopes and expectations of therapeutic outcomes, (c) orientation to the cognitive model, (d) setting out a plan of action, and (e) getting feedback from Frank regarding the session.

More specifically, the initial sessions with Frank would focus on our striving to fully understand his worldview. How does Frank view himself, his environment, and his future? If Frank identifies his aggressiveness as a focus of treatment, then Herpertz and Sass (1997) advocate for a detailed assessment of the aggressive acts, their antecedents, and accompanying cognitions as well as emotions, and finally their consequences.

Using the "Life Review" technique developed by Young (2002b), we could immediately begin working on Frank's schema. As such, we could elicit information from Frank that would provide evidence from his history that supports and contradicts his schema. The goal in this case is first to help Frank appreciate how his schemas direct his perceptions and feelings, thereby rigidly maintaining the schema. A second focus would be to help Frank assess the value and purpose of maintaining a particular schema or schema set.

Based on the fact that Frank is being court-ordered into treatment, it is expected that he will be somewhat reluctant to fully participate in therapy. Therefore, it may be more valuable to begin with more behavioral rather than cognitive techniques. Frank may be more inclined to accept more concrete behavioral techniques that don't seem as much like "psychobabble." Although cognitive exercises would serve to weaken Frank's schema, core beliefs may still be triggered in specific situations, causing the patient to continue behaving in ways that reinforce the schema. This further reinforces the need for using behavioral exercises in conjunction with cognitive exercises (when Frank is ready) to further challenge thoughts and behavior.

Behavioral Pattern-Breaking is a technique where Frank would be encouraged to stop behaving in ways that reinforce his schema. Understanding that Frank's primary schemas are (a) "My happiness/pleasure is paramount" and (b) "I can't count on anyone else, I have to do what's right for me," the therapist could set up behavioral experiments where Frank could test out the expectations that his behaviors will result in specified outcomes. Since Frank's lack of self-control can be at least partially explained by his schema, self-control training may be more likely to work if it is understood that the delay of gratification is paired with the appropriate consumption of gratification (Strayhorn, 2002b). It is further suggested that reinforcement be contingent on the accomplishment of self-control tasks.

Frank would also benefit from developing and improving his decision-making skills. As such, we might assist Frank with identifying "choice points," developing and listing alternative options, predicting consequences, and utilizing all that information in making a pro-social choice. Self-control by definition, is choosing and enacting a better but less pleasurable option; but if the person does not generate the better options, the pleasure principle is likely to be the default (Strayhorn, 2002b). Another step toward greater self-control would be in Frank's ability to self-monitor his behavior. Frank's impulsiveness has been identified as a major obstacle. Strayhorn suggests that failure to monitor one's own behavior is often a cause of failure of self-control.

A question that we would raise regarding Frank's impulsiveness is whether he might become so fanatically preoccupied with obtaining something that he believes that he wants, needs, or is entitled to that he becomes determined to have "it" by whatever means necessary? If this is the case, then there may be something to be said in regard to the "balance between too little and too much attention to the forbidden fruit" (Strayhorn, 2002b).

> Psychological techniques for managing anger are useful for patients who are able to tolerate a therapeutic environment and to discuss their own behavior. The key issue is to identify triggering situations and the automatic patterns of thought that precede an outburst of aggression. (Marlowe & Sugarman, 1997).

Homework is also a very important aspect of CBT that would have to be reinforced and shaped with Frank. Because there are 168 hours in a week, a one-hour session represents less than 1% of his week. Homework is very helpful for fighting schemas. "It keeps the work present in the patient's mind and helps to focus during the week on what has been accomplished during session" (Young, 2002, p. 218). "Just as a muscle is fatigued in the short run but strengthened in the long run by exercise, so self-control skills may be strengthened by exercising them and practicing them" (Strayhorn, 2002a).

8. Are there special cautions to be observed in working with this patient? Are there any particular resistances you would expect, and how would you deal with them?

Based on Frank's history of aggressive behavior, it is likely that we will experience this style of behavior emerging during treatment. When working with patients with ASPD it is not uncommon for there to be episodes of violence, threats to staff, and overall disruption of the clinical milieu (Cawthra & Gibb, 1998). "The sensitive nature of the relationship means that the therapist must exercise great caution in working with individuals with personality disorders. Few patients test the patience and determination of the therapist more than the Axis II group" (Freeman & Jackson, 1998, p. 331).

In formulating a treatment plan, we would explicitly inform Frank about his diagnosis of Antisocial Personality Disorder and set clear requirements for his involvement in treatment. Otherwise, he is not likely to see any reason or purpose in continuing psychotherapy other than for the fact that he is court-ordered. We do not think that it will be a surprise for Frank to learn his diagnosis. It would be useless to get into a debate concerning the diagnosis, but it would help him to understand that this is a categorization. It makes it even simpler to demonstrate that by changing certain aspects of his behavior, he can in fact alter the diagnosis.

9. Are there any areas that you would choose to avoid or not address with this patient, and why?

Based on the importance of forming a collaborative partnership with Frank, we would work to not avoid issues. The avoidance of so many issues in his life has added up to the present circumstance. Rather we would endeavor to be flexible and creative with how certain issues are raised. Similarly, educating Frank about his schema and how these beliefs impact his behavior would be an important factor to consider. From Young's perspective, it is essential to explain the nature of Early Maladaptive Schemas, domains, processes, and modes to the patient in order to develop a shared understanding of the problems and core issues involved (Young, 2002, p. 212).

10. Is medication warranted for this patient? What effect would you hope/expect for this medication to have?

"A combination of genetic or organic factors create that pattern of neurophysiology that includes remarkably low threat-arousal, with consequent thrill seeking and impulsivity" (Ochman, 1999). According to Robinson (2003, p. 67), there are two potential areas for a psychopharmacological approach with Frank. These include: 1) the reduction of impulsivity and 2) the reduction of angry outbursts. Selective Serotonin Reuptake Inhibitors (SSRIs) as well as some mood stabilizers have been shown to have some success with these target behaviors (Robinson, p. 67). These medications have demonstrated effectiveness with delaying gratification and decreasing impulsivity in animal studies (Strayhorn, 2002a).

Findings by Soderstrom, Blennow, Sjodin, and Forsman, (2003) suggest that aggression may be related to a high dopamine turnover in combination with a relative serotonergic dysregulation (leading to disinhibition of aggressive impulses). "Given this background, dopamine modulating drugs, alone or in combination with serotonin reuptake inhibitors (or drugs with combined dopamine and serotonin modulating action), might be of interest in treatment of aggressive psychopathy" (Soderstrom et al.). A study by Oldham (1994) demonstrated that symptomatic improvement can be achieved by targeted psychopharmacology. Medications such as Lithium, Carbamazepine, and SSRIs that have an impulse-stabilizing effect can be used for impulsive dyscontrol.

However, this issue may be a moot point. Due to Frank's worldview, he believes that the rest of the world is screwed up for not accepting him the way he is. It is therefore unlikely that he would agree to a trial of medications, nor do we believe that he is likely to comply with a medication regimen on an ongoing basis. It may, in fact, become a point of contention and resistance. There will be enough of that to go around!

11. What are the strengths of the patient that can be used in the therapy?

Certainly Frank's intelligence, creativity, and energy can all be used in the therapy. We might capsule our goals in this regard as trying to use the pathology in the service of the therapy. Frank takes challenges very seriously. If he were told that very few people with his problem stay in therapy or make life changes, we might appeal to his competitive style to "beat the system." His verbal ability will be useful as long as we are not drawn into debates on philosophical issues ("Just what is the meaning of good and evil?"), societal problems ("What would you expect of someone raised in my neighborhood?"), or cultural stereotypes ("He is nothing but a pushy Jew").

12. How would you address limits, boundaries, and limit setting with this patient?

It would be particularly important for us to model appropriate behavior and to maintain firm boundaries and limits. Furthermore, a clear understanding must be maintained and reinforced in regard to Frank living within the rules of society. A consistent approach, delivered within realistic limits, is paramount. Time should be taken to assure that Frank has a full understanding of what services can be delivered, by whom, in what time period, and what outcomes could be expected. "It is important in any therapeutic interaction to outline the limits and expected behavior of the therapist and patient: however, this is essential with ASPD patients, due to their generally poor sense of boundaries" (Beck et al., 2004, p. 169).

Frank would undoubtedly test the limits of our therapeutic relationship. Given his history it should go without saying that attempting to develop a relationship with someone who has difficulties forming relationships is a challenging and often daunting task (Marlowe & Sugarman, 1997). Nevertheless, the aim should be in developing a stable, long-term relationship with Frank.

It is recommended that therapists clearly outline and adhere to the pre-arranged length of the session, the policy on session cancellation, the rules about between-session contacts, the homework requirement, and appropriate use of the emergency phone number. The treatment contract should include an agreed-on number of sessions and expected behavioral change. The therapist must make sure that the patient is socialized or educated to the CBT model. To make sure that there is appropriate informed consent for therapy, the therapist must explain what the therapy involves, the goals and plans of the therapy, the importance of therapeutic collaboration, the particular areas of difficulty that will be emphasized, and the likely techniques that will be used in therapy (Freeman & Jackson, 1998, p. 328).

Therapists, especially those working with personality-disordered individuals, must be able to create boundaries between their professional and nonprofessional life. Using leisure activities and continually seeking feedback from colleagues are key features in providing the necessary relief from work and preventing burnout (Beck et al., 2004, p. 170).

13. Would you want to involve significant others in therapy? Would you use out-of-session work (homework) with this patient? What would you use?

The identifying features of ASPD are more clearly found in Frank's history than in the interview. Antisocial individuals will often minimize parts of their histories that would otherwise incriminate or inconvenience them, either with outright lies or with rationalization and a subtle choice of words (Reid, 2001). The history should not be limited to the patient's comments, but should include as many other resources as available.

Significant others may provide a different source of revealing information on the patient's current functioning and past behavior (Beck et al., 2004, p. 167). "The patient's significant others can be invaluable allies in the therapeutic endeavor by helping the patient to do homework and reality testing, and by offering support in making changes" (Freeman & Jackson, 1998, p. 331). Any previous psychological testing, school records, court evaluations, or medical records should be available. The more that we know, the better.

Homework would consist of self-monitoring of dysfunctional thoughts and engaging in behavioral experiments aimed at challenging dysfunctional thoughts and, in some cases, enhancing specific social skills.

14. What would be the issues to be addressed in termination? How would termination and relapse prevention be structured?

There would be a number of important factors to consider regarding relapse prevention with Frank. First of all, the chronic, inflexible nature of personality disorders must always be kept in mind. Frank would need to build a collection of relapse prevention strategies. They would be framed as, "If 'A' happens, I do 'B' to cope with it. If 'C' happens, I do 'D.' " The fewer choices that Frank has, the better. Throughout therapy we would focus on his effectively coping with the various stressors in his life. It would be important to prime Frank for setbacks. Frank should be instructed to avoid all-or-nothing thinking, in order to reduce the feeling of failure at the first sign of a lapse.

The concept of "momentum" is key to any relapse prevention program. There is validity to the notion of "being on a roll" or "falling off the wagon": self-control or self-indulgence seems to acquire momentum. The dieter or the alcoholic, after eating a bowl of ice cream or drinking a glass of wine, thinks, 'I've already broken my rule; I might as well break it in a big way,' and proceeds to go on a binge (Strayhorn, 2002a).

An issue that would concern us with Frank is the fact that he might learn to master the language of therapy, learning which responses signal positive change. He might learn what he thinks he is supposed to say, how he is supposed to feel, and how he is supposed to act in order to demonstrate to us (or other authorities) that he has made marked improvement (Davis-Barron, 1995). Since Frank sees nothing wrong with his attitude or behavior, he will likely see no need to change, yet he may be astutely aware of what he needs to do to convince us that he has changed.

15. What do you see as the hoped for mechanisms of change for this patient?

There are two essential mechanisms for change that are addressed in Frank's case. First and foremost are his schemas. If his schemas are altered, even slightly, his behavior and affect would, ideally, follow. For example, Frank's schema of not being able to count on an inconsistent and abusive parent may have been both functional and protective as he was growing up; however his schema has long since outlived its usefulness as Frank became an adult. This is a point that must be made again and again in the course of the therapy.

The second target of change would be in Frank's interpersonal behaviors and his relationships. Understanding the root causes of antisocial activity is important because it allows the therapist to plan treatment strategies that target these key areas for change. "Without an adequate understanding of the underlying etiology, prevention and treatment are likely to be ineffective because they may target the wrong mechanisms of change" (Brinkley et al., 2004).

Relationships serve as the context for the development of emotional regulation (an important aspect of self control). Improvement in patients with Antisocial Personality Disorder (perhaps the quintessence of self-control problems) is predicted by the ability of such patients to form working relationships with a therapist (Strayhorn, 2002b).

Furthermore, as mentioned previously in this chapter, establishing the baseline severity of Frank's characterological disorder would be essential when assessing change in his core personality. Psychotherapy will not realistically cure his dysfunction. "The cruder dichotomous measure of presence or absence of the disorder does not allow any consideration of amelioration of dysfunction. Change may be difficult to assess if only looking at the presence or absence of a personality disorder" (Norton & Dolan, 1995). People with Antisocial Personality Disorder have been shown to learn from experience when the contingencies are immediate, well-specified, tangible, and personally relevant (Beck et al., 2004, p. 163). Although it would most likely be a long road toward behavioral change, hope is not lost on Frank, nor on the therapist with the courage and stamina to tackle such a difficult case.

REFERENCES

American Psychiatric Association. (2000). *Diagnostic and statistical manual of mental disorders* (4th revised ed.). Washington DC: Author.

Beck, A., Freeman, A., Davis, D., & Associates. (2004). *Cognitive therapy of personality disorders* (2nd ed.). New York: Guilford Press.

Beck, A., Rush, A., Shaw, B., & Emery, G. (1979). Cognitive therapy of depression. New York: Guilford Press

Brinkley, C. A., Newman, J. P., Widiger, T. A., & Lynam, D. R. (2004). Two approaches to parsing the heterogeneity of psychopathy. *Clinical Psychology, 11*(1), 69–94.

Cawthra, R., & Gibb, R. (1998). Severe personality disorder—whose responsibility? *British Journal of Psychiatry, 173*(7), 8–10.

Davis-Barron, S. (1995). Psychopathic patients pose dilemma for physicians and society [special report]. *Canadian Medical Association Journal, 152*(8), 1314–1317.

Freeman, A., & Jackson, J. (1998). Cognitive behavioural treatment of personality disorders. In N. Tarrier, A. Wells, & G. Haddock (Eds.), *Treating complex cases: The cognitive behavioural therapy approach* (pp. 319–339). West Sussex, England: John Wiley & Sons.

Freeman, A., Pretzer, J., Fleming, B., & Simon, K. (1990). *Clinical applications of cognitive therapy.* New York: Plennum Press.

Freeman, A., Saxon-Hunt, M., & Yacono, L.Y. (2004). Cambios paralelos en psico-terapia para el terapeuta y el paciente con un trastorno de la personalidad (Parallel change in the therapist and the patient in the treatment of personality disorders). In V. E. Caballo (Ed.), *Manual de trastornos de la personalidad.* Madrid, Spain: Editorial Sinthesis.

Herpertz, S., & Sass, H. (1997). Psychopathy and antisocial syndromes. *Current Opinion in Psychiatry, 10*(6), 436–440.

Marlowe, M., & Sugarman, P. (1997). ABC of mental health: Disorders of personality, *British Medical Journal, 315*(7), 176–179.

Norton, K., & Dolan, B. (1995). Assessing change in personality disorder. *Current Opinion in Psychiatry, 8*(6), 371–375.

Ochman, F. M. (1999). Psychopathy: Antisocial, criminal, and violent behavior. *Journal of Nervous and Mental Disorders, 187*(5), 321–323.

Oldham, J. M. (1994). Personality disorders: Current perspectives [special communications]. *Journal of the American Medical Association, 272*(22), 1770–1776.

Perry, J., Banon, E., & Ianni, F. (1999). Effectiveness of psychotherapy for personality disorder [special articles]. *American Journal of Psychiatry, 156*(9), 1312–1321.

Persons, J. B. (1989), *Cognitive therapy in practice: A case formulation approach.* New York: W. W. Norton.

Reid, W. H. (2001). Antisocial personality, psychopathy, and forensic psychiatry. *Journal of Psychiatric Practice, 7*(1), 55–58

Robinson, D. J. (2003), *The personality disorders explained* (2nd ed.). Port Huron, MI: Rapid Psychler Press.

Roy, S., & Tyrer, P. (2001). Treatment of personality disorders. *Current Opinion in Psychiatry, 14*(6), 555–558.

Soderstrom, H., Blennow, K., Sjodin, A-K., & Forsman, A. (2003). New evidence for an association between the CFS HVA:5—HIAA ratio and psychopathic traits. *Neurology, Neurosurgery, & Psychiatry, 74*(7), 918–921.

Strayhorn, J. M. (2002a). Self-control: Theory and research. *Child and Adolescent Psychiatry, 41*(1), 7–16.

Strayhorn, J. M. (2002b). Self-control: Toward systematic training programs. *Child and Adolescent Psychiatry, 41*(1), 17–27.

Young, J. E. (1994). *Cognitive therapy for personality disorders: A schema focused approach* (revised ed.). Sarasota, FL: Professional Resource Press.

Young, J. E. (2003). Schema-focused therapy for personality disorders. In G. Simos (Ed.), *Cognitive behaviour therapy: A guide for the practicing clinician* (pp. 201–222). New York: Taylor & Francis.

CHAPTER 8

Dialectical Behavior Therapy

Robin A. McCann, Katherine Anne Comtois, and Elissa M. Ball

Describe your treatment model.

Dialectical Behavior Therapy (DBT) is a comprehensive and structured behavior therapy. It has been found to be effective in randomized trials with suicidal women diagnosed with Borderline Personality Disorder (Lieb, Zanarini, Schmahl, Linehan, & Bohus, 2004; Linehan, 1993) and substance-using women diagnosed with Borderline Personality Disorder (Linehan et al., 1999). Nonrandomized trials suggest potential with other complex, difficult to treat patients including: forensic inpatients (McCann & Ball, 1996), juvenile offenders (Trupin, Stewart, Beach, & Boesky, in press), batterers (Fruzzetti & Levensky, 2000), and suicidal adolescents (Miller, Rathus, Leigh, & Landsman, 1996). Randomized trials are currently underway to test the effectiveness of DBT with correctional populations (Berzins & Trestman, 2004).

Comprehensive DBT targets the client's motivation to engage in effective behavior, provides skills training, and assures skills generalization. DBT's structure is based on a biosocial theory and includes articulated treatment stages and targets, flexible treatment modalities, and many treatment strategies. The two major treatment strategies, validation and problem solving, are balanced by dialectics.

Comprehensive DBT delivers therapy in four modes: Individual Therapy, Group Skills Training, Case Consultation, and Phone Calls. Each mode has it own set of targets (see Table 8.1). For example, should therapy-interfering behavior (see question 1) occur in Skills Training, the Skills Trainer refers such behavior to the individual therapist. Such referral enables the Skills Trainer

TABLE 8.1
DBT Modes & Targets

Mode	Target
Individual Therapy	Decrease life-threatening, therapy-interfering behaviors, and quality-of-life-interfering behaviors
Group Skills Training	Increase skill acquisition & rehearsal
Phone Calls	Decrease life-threatening behaviors. Increase skills generalization
Case Consultation	Increase DBT adherence. Decrease therapist burnout

to stay on task with their primary target: skills acquisition. The individual therapist is generally responsible for phone calls. Importantly, the function of phone calls is to assess risk and prompt skills generalization, not to provide therapy. Thus a frequent opening line for the therapist during phone calls is "Open your skills training book."

The typical structure of the individual therapy session is as follows:

1. Review self-monitoring log (called DBT Diary Card).
2. Set agenda from information provided on the DBT Diary Card (e.g. life-threatening behaviors first, therapy-interfering before quality-of-life interfering, etc.).
3. Complete a Behavioral and Solution Analysis on target behavior.
4. Role-play skills identified in Behavioral Analysis.

The function of the Skills Training group is to teach and practice skills. Skills are organized into the following modules: Core Mindfulness, Distress Tolerance, Emotion Regulation, and Interpersonal Effectiveness (Linehan, 1993b).

The function of the Case Consultation Meeting is to keep the therapist on task (DBT) and prevent burnout. Biosocial theory and DBT assumptions structure the therapist's behavior in Case Consultation. See question 4 for examples of DBT assumptions.

Biosocial theory as originally conceptualized by Marsha Linehan hypothesizes that Borderline Personality Disorder (BPD) is the result of a transaction between a biological dysfunction in the emotion regulation system and an invalidating environment. Individuals with BPD are thought to be particularly emotionally vulnerable and therefore more sensitive to environmental invalidation.

Frank is clearly not emotionally vulnerable. Rather he appears emotionally insensitive and may meet criteria for Psychopathy (as measured by the Hare Psychopathy Checklist–Revised). McCann, Ball, & Ivanoff (2000) extended biosocial theory to emotionally insensitive individuals such as Frank. Emotionally insensitive individuals have difficulties processing and understanding emotional material (Hare, 2003). They have lower emotional arousal to distressing images and fail to demonstrate differential responses between neutral versus Emotion-laden lexical tasks (Hare). Mr. J's failure to express either sadness or fear as a child appears to be an example of lower arousal or emotional insensitivity that is perhaps biological in etiology. Biosocial theory as extended to such emotionally insensitive individuals suggests that antisocial personality disorder (ASPD) may result from the transaction of emotional insensitivity with invalidation over time.

But what is invalidation? Invalidating responses include neglect, disregard, direct criticism, and punishment (Linehan, 1993). Such environments indiscriminately reject expression of feelings and intermittently reinforce escalation of emotional responses. Invalidating environments of individuals with ASPD are characterized by frequent experience and witnessing of physical abuse (Waltz, Babcock, Jacobson, & Gottman, 2000), harsh & inconsistent discipline, and inadequate supervision (Patterson, DeBaryshe, & Ramsey, 1989). Emotional insensitivity may transact with invalidation in two ways. First, there is evidence that parents of antisocial children ignore or inappropriately respond to pro-social behavior (Patterson et al.). Second, antisocial peers reinforce antisocial behavior (Patterson et al.).

The DBT model starts with a dialectical balance of the two major DBT treatment strategies: Validation and Change. Validating difficult–to-treat patients, without pushing for change, results in failure to learn anything new. Pushing difficult-to-treat patients to change, without validation, results in patients feeling highly aroused, which prevents them from learning anything new. Such invalidation, in transaction with emotion dysregulation, may maintain Borderline Personality Disorder (Linehan, 1993) and Antisocial Personality Disorder (McCann et al., 2000). Validation promotes change by decreasing client arousal, thereby increasing the client's ability to learn something new. Validation helps "the medicine go down." Here the "medicine" includes change strategies such as behavioral analysis, skills training, contingency management, exposure therapy, and cognitive modification (Linehan, 1993a).

A dialectical position in DBT also informs the biosocial theory and balances treatment strategies, skills, and assumptions. DBT assumes both that "patients are doing the best they can" and assumes that "patients may not have caused all of their own problems, but they have to solve them anyway" (Linehan, 1993). DBT includes both Change and Acceptance skills. DBT teaches patients skills to change their emotions (Emotion Regulation

Skills) and to change their environment (Interpersonal Effectiveness Skills). DBT also teaches patients skills to accept reality (Mindfulness) and crises (Distress Tolerance) without making situations worse. For example, it may be useful for Frank to mindfully accept that he is not "always in control of every situation." He may need Distress Tolerance distraction skills to decrease his impulsivity during crises, such as the failure of the Land Development Company. Lying to his wife, taking bets from racetrack junkies, and drinking caused a bad situation (losing his company) to become worse (losing his wife and gaining additional charges). Similarly, the DBT therapist balances both acceptance and change. On the one hand the therapist validates Frank: "Of course you felt ashamed!" On the other hand the therapist pushes Frank for change: "Drinking is your mortal enemy! Let's figure out the 100 other ways you can cope with shame!"

A dialectical worldview assumes that change is constant and transactional (Linehan, 1993a). In other words, it is assumed that even a client who meets criteria for Psychopathy will change—given the right combination of new skills and environmental contingencies.

1. What would be your therapeutic goal? What is the primary goal? The secondary goal?

Forensic treatment must target violent recidivism (Hodgins, 2002). Cognitive behavioral treatments are more effective in reducing recidivism than less structured therapies (Wong & Hare, 1998). DBT is a cognitive-behavioral treatment that targets life-threatening behaviors. Thus, the primary goal is obtaining Frank's commitment to decrease behaviors that are life-threatening to others—that is, bar brawls, assaults, using snakes to intimidate, and threats to kill. No commitment, no DBT. Importantly, DBT therapists do not label patients as "amotivated" or "resistant." It is the DBT therapist's job to sell and shape commitment. Again, this is a dialectic between demands for change (i.e., making and acting on a commitment) versus acceptance (i.e., assuming making such a commitment is hard and assistance is needed to make and maintain it). For example, the DBT therapist might sell decreasing life-threatening behaviors by linkage to Mr. J's intrinsic goals: maintaining his relationship with his wife, getting off probation, avoiding incarceration, etc. Given Mr. J's anti-authority values, it will be helpful to stress his freedom to choose or reject DBT and the concomitant absence of viable alternatives. So the DBT therapist might say something like "You are free to commit to decreasing life-threatening behaviors. You are free to commit to continuing life-threatening behaviors. If you commit to decreasing life-threatening behaviors we can begin DBT. If you commit to continuing life-threatening behaviors we cannot begin DBT and it is reasonable to assume that such a commitment would incur concern from your probation officer."

DBT structures treatment by Level of Disorder (Linehan, 1993):

Level 1: Behavioral Dyscontrol
Level 2: Quiet Desperation
Level 3: Problems in Living
Level 4: Incompleteness

Mr. J's behavior reflects Level 1: Behavioral Dyscontrol. The primary treatment goal is behavioral control or self-management. Self-management is wholly consistent with expert recommendations regarding the treatment of Psychopathy (Wong & Hare; 1998).

DBT targets are hierarchically organized in order of importance as shown in Table 8.2. After obtaining commitment to stop life-threatening behaviors, the next goal is to start changing this behavior, specifically stopping Mr. J's physical violence and behaviors closely related to physical violence. Examples of behaviors closely related to violence include: homicide/assault-related expectancies & beliefs (e.g., "Shut up or you are dead!" or "He deserves what he got!") and homicide/assault-related affects (e.g., intense shame).

Mr. J meets criteria for ASPD, he may meet criteria for Psychopathy, and he evidences therapy-interfering behaviors during assessment. Decreasing therapy-interfering behaviors is the secondary goal. In this case, therapy-interfering behaviors might include non-collaborative behaviors such as: denying responsibility, refusing to sign releases, and blaming others. Therapy-interfering behaviors may include behaviors that push therapists' limits

TABLE 8.2
DBT Stage 1 Target Hierarchy

Decrease

    Life-threatening behaviors toward self or others

    Therapy-interfering behaviors

    Quality-of-life-interfering behaviors

Increase

    Mindfulness

    Interpersonal effectiveness

    Emotion regulation

    Distress tolerance

    Self-Management

or reduce their motivation to treat: disdain and an icy cold glare or a manner that induces fear or humiliation. Without resolution of therapy-interfering behaviors, therapy will end prior to achieving the primary goal: decreasing aggression. The third DBT goal or target is quality-of-life-interfering behaviors, including Frank's substance abuse, ineffective work skills, non-violent illegal activities, and property damage. Note that Frank's poor work skills and substance use are dynamic risk factors which may increase recidivism (Andrews & Bonta, 1998).

After commitment, it is expected that Frank's behavior will be intermittently inconsistent. It is normal for people to maintain a variable state of commitment (e.g., to exercise, diet, etc.) (Miller & Rollnick, 2002). The DBT therapist is cognizant that re-commitment is necessary over and over again. The DBT therapist will ask Frank to re-commit to decreasing life-threatening and therapy-interfering behaviors, over and over and over—each time linking such a commitment to Mr. J's personal goals and providing skills that make commitment easier to maintain.

2. What further information would you want to have to assist in structuring this patient's treatment? Are their specific assessment tools you would use? What would be the rationale for using these tools?

Three types of assessments are needed. First, an assessment of static and dynamic risk is mandatory. Intense psychotherapeutic intervention is correlated with decreased recidivism in high-risk cases and correlated with increased recidivism in low-risk cases (Andrews & Bonta, 1998). Frank's charm, lying, lack of remorse or empathy, shallow affect, aggressive outbursts, and irresponsibility suggest the possibility of Psychopathy, a static risk factor. A high Psychopathy score suggests high risk and intense intervention. Treatment must be adapted to account for Mr. J's Psychopathy (Andrews & Bonta). For example, DBT emotion regulation skills are adapted to account for his relative emotional insensitivity (McCann et al., 2000).

Frank's dynamic risk factors or criminogenic needs must be assessed. Criminogenic needs are those treatment targets that are closely linked to violent or criminal behavior (Andrews & Bonta, 1998). Dynamic risk factors, unlike static risk factors, can change with therapeutic intervention (Wong & Gordon, 2000). A measure of dynamic risk, such as the Violence Risk Scale (Wong & Gordon), might identify the following dynamic risk factors: criminal personality, poor work ethic, interpersonal aggression, poor insight into aggression, substance abuse, antisocial beliefs (e.g., blames others, justifies antisocial behavior, pro-violence sentiments, etc.), poor self-management, and a deteriorating marital relationship. DBT directly targets interpersonal aggression, self-management, and substance abuse. DBT indirectly targets anti-social beliefs and marital relationships through its emphasis on the acquisition of pro-social skills (see Interpersonal Effectiveness module) and emotion regulation. Given Mr. J's likely high Psychopathy score, such pro-social skills must be linked to his self-interest.

The second type of assessment needed is idiographic behavioral assessment. Each episode of life-threatening, therapy-interfering, or any other target behavior must be assessed with a behavioral analysis. A behavioral analysis is composed of "links" including triggers, contextual factors, vulnerability factors, and consequences. Such "links" may include: environmental events and Frank's thoughts, feelings, body sensations, and actions. See queston 7 for discussion of behavioral analysis.

The third assessment is psychiatric. The Case Study suggests that Bipolar Disorder and Schizophrenia have been ruled out. Nevertheless, Frank's moodiness, irritability, impulsivity, and so forth, suggest that it is important to rule-out other psychiatric disorders. ASPD co-occurs with major axis I disorders. For example, in a sample of 107 inmates carrying Psychotic or Major Depression diagnoses, 71 carried a concomitant ASPD diagnosis (Hodgins & Cote, 1993). Regardless of the presence of other psychiatric disorders, medications may be effective in reducing Frank's impulsivity, moodiness, and irritability.

3. What is your conceptualization of this patient's personality, behavior, affective state, and cognitions?

A series of behavioral analyses must be completed to conceptualize Frank's case. These analyses will identify the controlling variables for his life-threatening and other target behaviors (see question 7). However, we might hypothesize the following.

Frank's aggression developed and is maintained by his (biological) emotional insensitivity and by his environmental modeling and negative reinforcement. Fearing his temper, parental figures and siblings avoided intervening in Mr. J's early antisocial behavior. Frank's wife also avoids confronting him. Frank's father is clearly a model for his aggressive behavior.

DBT conceptualizes problems as a disorder in the emotion regulation system. There is some evidence that, while Frank is emotionally insensitive to others, he is vulnerable to shame (or humiliation). While both shame and guilt are "moral" emotions, there are important distinctions. Guilty people worry about their effect on others, and wish to confess, apologize, or repair. Frank clearly does not feel guilty! Humiliated people worry about themselves, hide, escape, and most importantly, strike back (Tangney & Dearing, 2002).

Shamed individuals bolster themselves by directing their hostility toward others. Frank appears to feel shame.

Shame is negatively correlated with empathy and positively correlated with psychopathology (Tangney & Dearing, 2002). Should shame function as a controlling variable for aggression, Frank's treatment might include: (a) accepting shame, (b) breaking the link between shame and anger, (c) breaking the link between shame and aggression through informal exposure therapy, and (d) teaching Frank confession and repair skills, thereby increasing his focus on others.

4. What potential pitfalls would you envision in this therapy? What would the difficulties be and what would you envision being the sources of these difficulties?

The therapist's failure to identify therapy-interfering behaviors and observe her/his limits will decrease commitment and ultimately destroy therapy. Frank is court-ordered to treatment; involuntary treatment may exacerbate therapy-interfering behaviors, notably behaviors that push therapists' limits. For instance, the assessment interview suggests that Frank will likely act in ways to induce fear or humiliation in the therapist. Such feelings will decrease therapist commitment and may evoke therapy-interfering behavior from the therapist (e.g., use of coercive power). The therapist must address such behavior directly. For example, "Frank, questions to me such as 'Why don't you make believe you have a life of your own?' erode my motivation to do a good job with you. My doing a good job is essential in your getting off probation. Stop asking such questions." The therapist will conduct a behavioral analysis of the controlling variables for the behavior (examples might be anger and shame regarding court-ordered treatment), and provide and reinforce the use of specific alternative behaviors. For example, "So, could we agree that in the future when you have the urge to be threatening or nasty, you will instead use a distraction skill such as thoughts (counting breath, tiles, thoughts, etc.)." When the needed strategies are not clear to the therapist or not working as well as one had hoped, regular case consultation with the DBT team targets the problem, analyzes it with the therapist, generates solutions, teaches the therapist new skills or provides opportunities to practice skills, and reinforces the therapist for sticking with the DBT model and remaining dialectical with the patient.

DBT structures therapy with treatment Assumptions and the Target Behavior Hierarchy. The DBT therapist who accepts such assumptions will more probably enjoy, and thus be committed to, working with Frank. On the one hand, DBT therapists accept that Frank is "doing the best he can" (Linehan,

1993). In other words, given his learning history and current contingencies, his aggressive and humiliating behavior makes sense. Importantly this DBT assumption is dialectically balanced by the following corollary: Frank "must learn new behaviors in all relevant contexts" (Linehan, 1993). In other words, while Frank's aggression makes sense, he must decrease aggression and increase effective interpersonal skills with everyone, everywhere, at all times, on or off probation.

DBT also structures therapy with the Target Hierarchy. Life-threatening behavior is the only Stage 1 target more important than therapy-interfering behaviors. Therapy-interfering behaviors are behaviors that interfere with the provision or reception of therapy. The source of such therapy-interfering behaviors is the transaction between the client and the therapist. A transaction, unlike an interaction, is dynamic, changing both the client and the therapist. Thus, patients like Frank are called "butterfly" clients because they fail to attend therapy, fail to attach in therapy, fail to pay attention, and so forth. Such butterfly clients can transact with therapists, turning the therapist into a "butterfly" therapist (Dimeff, Rizvi, Brown, & Linehan, 2000). In other words, patients shape therapists to become bad therapists. For example, it is expected that Frank will blame the therapist for his problem. Such behavior could shape the therapist to blame Frank in return. So DBT therapists observe their limits by stating: "When you blame me I don't particularly want to help you. Please stop blaming me. Your job is to act in a manner so that I want to help you."

Unresolved dialectical dilemmas in treatment are a source of therapy-interfering behaviors. On the one hand the DBT therapist helps patients change in ways that bring them closer to their own ultimate goals (Linehan, 1993). On the other hand, the therapist has a legal role as an advisor to the court. Such a role has potential for coercion. Intra-role conflict, for example conflict between security and therapeutic roles, is correlated with burnout (Allard, Wortley, & Stewart, 2003). Clarification of roles is mandatory. For example, treatment may target drug abstinence and drug abstinence will likely be a parole condition. On the one hand, Frank failing to report substance use to the therapist is therapy-interfering. On the other hand, the therapist reporting Frank's substance use to Probation is also therapy-interfering. Open discussion of this tricky dialectical dilemma is essential.

5. To what level of coping would you see this patient reaching as an immediate result of therapy? What result would be long term subsequent to the ending of therapy?

Should Frank commit to DBT, it is expected that Frank would complete his probation, thereby avoiding prison, thereby increasing his odds of achieving "a life worth living." In regard to long-term results, on the one hand DBT is "empirically minded" treatment and thus reluctant, in the absence of empirically validated predictors, to predict long-term results (Fruzzetti & Levensky, 2000). On the other hand, there is ample evidence attesting to the effectiveness of cognitive behavioral treatments with correctional populations (Andrews & Bonta, 1998). Several randomized studies are underway examining the effectiveness of DBT with correctional populations (Berzins & Trestman, 2004).

However, it can be hypothesized that successful completion of DBT would result in a decrease in criminogenic risk factors such as impulsivity, homicide and assault expectancies and emotions, and substance abuse. Such decreases would hypothetically be associated with increases in occupational stability, a factor at least modestly associated with decreases in recidivism (Bogue, 2002).

6. What would be your timeline? What would be the frequency and duration of the sessions?

The time line for reducing Stage 1 targets (gaining control of dysregulated behavior) is 1 year. The therapist will ask Frank to commit to 1 year of weekly 1-hour individual therapy sessions and 2.5 hours of weekly skills training sessions.

While Frank has a significant trauma history, it is possible that he does not need Stage 2 treatment: decreasing desperation and increasing emotional experiencing. First, there is no compelling evidence that emotional experiencing is a criminogenic need (McCann, Ivanoff, Beach, & Schmidt, in press). Second, perhaps because of his emotional insensitivity, Stage 2 treatment may not be needed. In other words, despite his trauma history, Frank does not appear emotionally desperate and may not need trauma work.

After completion of basic DBT, an advanced DBT skills group would be offered to Frank. Such an advanced group consists of DBT therapists shaping clients in setting the agenda, completing behavioral and solution analyses, and role-play of skills.

7. Are there specific techniques you would implement in the therapy? What would they be?

Repeated behavioral or "chain" analyses of specific incidents are necessary to understand and then decrease Frank's life-threatening, therapy-interfering, and quality-of-life-interfering behaviors. For example, the therapist would complete a behavioral or "chain" analysis of each of Frank's bar brawls.

Such analyses help determine the controlling variables for problem behaviors. Simplistically, this means that we determine whether the behavior is a function of cues (triggers) or consequences. Repeated chain analyses assess dysfunctional "links" including vulnerability factors, triggers, and consequences of the targeted behaviors. A link is presumed to be dysfunctional if it leads to behaviors inconsistent with Frank's long-term goals. For example, blaming others may provide short-term relief, but is inconsistent with Mr. J's presumed long-term goals: avoiding prison and ending probation.

Importantly, a dysfunctional link suggests solutions, that is, alternative behaviors. For example, a problem link such as blaming others suggests a variety of solutions. The therapist and patient work on the problem behavior over and over and over again, like water over a rock. Blaming others may be a function of skills deficits. Frank may lack mindfulness "Describe" skills (Linehan, 1993b): the ability to objectively and nonjudgmentally describe events, actions, and feelings. He may lack repair skills: apologizing and overcorrecting. Conversely, Frank may have the skills, but "lack motivation." For example, cues or consequences may maintain blaming behavior. Given childhood punishment, conflict may have become a cue for blaming behavior. Blaming may effectively help Frank escape from aversive consequences, an example of negative reinforcement. Fearful, others may provide positive reinforcement for his blaming.

Based on the behavior and solution analysis, one or two alternative behaviors to blaming are selected and agreed upon. This is followed by skills rehearsal and role-play of those alternate behaviors in circumstances mimicking those that trigger blaming behavior. Research suggests that skill rehearsal is critical in effective forensic treatment (Bogue, 2002). Attention is then paid to Mr. J's future behavior to be sure to reinforce shaping toward the alternative behavior and avoid future reinforcement of the ineffective behavior of blaming.

8. Are there special cautions to be observed in working with this patient? Are there any particular resistances you would expect, and how would you deal with them?

Yes, there is a special caution. It is easy to dislike Frank. Should Frank meet criteria for Psychopathy, there will be considerable reinforcement for therapists to predict poor outcome. Therapists may perceive lying, manipulation, and so forth, even when it is not present. Importantly, Frank may be proud to label himself as a bad guy or even a psychopath (Swann, Rentfrow, & Guinn, 2002). By glaring, humiliating others, and continuing criminal behavior, Frank will receive confirmation of his self-view: a bad guy! A therapist who merely accepts ("Yes, you are glaring because you are a psychopath!") maintains Frank's self-view. Conversely, a DBT therapist accepts (acknowledges) Mr. J's behavior, maybe even accepts the meaning of the behavior ("Yep, this is one of the behaviors that helps you meet criteria for psychopathy"), and yet consistently pushes for change ("Hey, quit giving me the evil eyeball!").

Case Consultation keeps the therapist on task and prevents burnout (Linehan, 1993a). It is unlikely that therapists will help Frank if they dislike or even hate him. Burnout is endemic to correctional settings and is more likely with difficult-to-treat patients (Maslach & Jackson, 1993) like Frank. Case Consultation meets (ideally) for 2 hours weekly and is structured in the following manner.

1. Mindfulness Practice
2. Agenda Setting
   a. Priority as per target hierarchy such as, life threatening first, and so on
   b. Therapist articulates what she wants:
      1. Problem Assessment
      2. Solution Assessment
      3. Validation
      4. Empathy for Patient

Problem assessment and empathy (for Frank) may be frequent consultation issues.

9. Are there any areas that you would choose to avoid or not address with this patient? Why?

No.

10. Is medication warranted for this patient? What effect would you hope/expect the medication to have?

There are no medications that treat Antisocial Personality Disorder directly. There are medications that can be helpful. Target symptoms that sometimes respond to medications in this group of patients include: irritability, impulsivity, thinking distortions, and anxiety.

Frank is not currently complaining of any of these symptoms. Until Frank identifies behaviors he would like to change, and he or his wife have developed the ability to observe and measure such problem behaviors, medication benefits would be unlikely. All medications have potential side-effects, and few patients are willing to tolerate these side-effects unless they can see clear benefits. None of the possible medications demonstrates enough efficacy to warrant obtaining a court order for the medication or asking the parole officer to require compliance as a condition of parole.

Possible classes of medications include: mood stabilizers, low dose atypical antipsychotics, and non-addictive anti-anxiety agents. The mood stabilizers can be useful in lowering a person's level of irritability and decreasing the tendency to act impulsively (Hollander et al., 2001). Frank certainly has problems with irritability and impulsive aggressive behavior, but the frequency appears relatively low. Therefore, it is unlikely that such a medication would be helpful enough to balance out expected side-effects. If Mr. J expressed an interest in a trial of such a medication, first choices would be valproic acid, oxycarbamazepine, or carbamazepine. These medications require less stringent blood level control than lithium. All have a significant likelihood of causing weight gain, which Frank would likely find intolerable, given his focus on his dress and physique. It is important that Frank and his wife self-monitor baseline ratings of irritability or edginess prior to a medication trial. Changes are likely to be subtle, such that lengthy baseline and follow-up measures would be important to assess benefit.

Benefit from a low dose atypical antipsychotic is somewhat more likely. Frank's early history with an abusive, demeaning father has likely resulted in frequent automatic antisocial cognitions, but it is unlikely that Frank recognizes these as cognitive distortions. Low dose antipsychotics appear to slow down the spontaneity and intensity of these thoughts, so that a patient can begin to observe and challenge their cognitions and control their reactions (Hollander et al., 2001; Zanarini & Frankenburg, 2001). It is unlikely that medications would provide much benefit unless the patient has begun to collaborate with a therapist to examine how his cognitions are linked to problem behaviors.

Typical antipsychotics such as haloperidol might be just as effective as atypical ones, but the risk-benefit ratio rules out these medications. Atypical antipsychotics such as risperidone, olanzepine, ziprazidone, quetiapine, and aripiprazole have many fewer side-effects and are therefore more likely to be acceptable to Frank. Possible sedation and weight gain are the side-effects most likely to be bothersome to a man with Antisocial Personality Disorder. Very small doses (0.5 mg risperidone, for example) may be effective without causing such side-effects. Such side-effects are unlikely with ziprazidone and aripiprazole, but these medications are much newer and have not yet been tested in this population. Theoretically, it would seem that they would be equally effective for cognitive distortions, but their lack of sedative properties and propensity to increase energy might be problematic.

Currently, Frank does not demonstrate problems with anxiety. Should such symptoms develop, and if medicating these symptoms seemed therapeutic, buspirone is often effective. In a man such as Frank who has both Antisocial Personality Disorder and a substance problem, benzodiazepines would be contraindicated because of their addictive potential.

11. What are the strengths of the patient that can be used in the therapy?

Frank has effective interpersonal effectiveness skills as evidenced by his ability to obtain jobs and charm others. However Frank needs to use his interpersonal skills in the service of his long-term goals, such as getting off probation and avoiding incarceration. Accessing "Wise Mind" or wisdom (Linehan, 1993) is essential for Frank. "Wise Mind," in Frank's case, means doing what is best not only for himself but for others.

12. How would you address limits, boundaries, and limit setting with this patient?

DBT therapists do not address boundaries. Boundaries are a psychodynamic concept and are not discussed in DBT, a cognitive-behavioral treatment. DBT therapists also do not set limits. Therapist limit setting implies that the patient has no limits, is amorphous. Such an implication is inconsistent with behavioral assumptions and laws.

DBT therapists do observe their personal limits, that is, they observe what patient behaviors they are willing or not willing to tolerate. DBT therapists honestly express or own these limits, before it is too late! "Too late" means that the therapist is ready to transfer the patient to someone else.

Behaviors that push therapist limits are called therapy-interfering behaviors, and these are second in importance only to life-threatening behaviors. Note that therapy-interfering behaviors are considered more important than quality-of-life-interfering behaviors: financial difficulties, criminal behaviors, unemployment, homelessness, and so forth!

Therapist limits are individualized, dynamic, and idiosyncratic. Such limits may include: phone call time/durations, therapist privacy, therapist time, aggressive behaviors (e.g., icy stares), and therapist willingness to treat such aggressive behavior. For example, it is not a DBT technique to tell

Frank that his "cold icy stare" is "inappropriate" or "hostile" or reflects his "poor boundaries." Conversely, it is a DBT technique to tell Frank "When you stare I don't like you. I can't help you if I don't like you. Please stop staring," or, more "radically genuine" (Linehan, 1997), "Hey Mr. J, stop giving me the evil eyeball!"

Importantly, Frank's "icy stare" might impinge on one and not on another therapist's limits. Limits are contextual, defined by space, time, and individuals' learning histories. Thus the therapist will, if necessary, extend or retract limits. So, for example, if Frank were physically injured, the therapist, who may generally observe "no touch" limits, might temporarily extend these limits. Conversely, if the therapist were giving birth, she certainly would not be expected to provide phone coaching to Frank! In this case, the therapist restricts her limits.

13. Would you want to involve significant others in the treatment? Would you use out of session work with this patient? What homework would you use?

Out of session homework is routine in cognitive behavioral treatments. DBT clients self-monitor feelings, urges to harm oneself and others, actions harming oneself and others, and skills use daily on a DBT Diary Card. Such self-monitoring induces reactivity and may change behavior in the desired direction (Watson & Tharp, 1977). The Diary Cards reflect the Stage 1 Target Hierarchy: life-threatening behaviors, and so forth (see question 1). The individual therapist reviews the DBT Diary Cards at the beginning of the session and uses the cards to structure the targets of the individual therapy session. For example, targeting life-threatening behaviors is a higher priority than quality-of-life-interfering behaviors. Additional homework is routine in DBT. The DBT individual therapist and client collaboratively determine additional homework assignments, which are frequently derived from solution analyses (see question 7). For example, should Frank wish to decrease anger, he might practice Acting Opposite to Anger (Linehan, 1993b) skills daily. If needed, Frank could borrow commercially developed tapes demonstrating these and other skills. In addition, Mr. J would be attending a weekly skills training group that will also assign weekly homework.

Involving significant others in treatment is ideal for the following reasons: (a) Significant others are a source of collateral data. (b) Teaching significant others skills may enhance patients' skills generalization. For example, teaching Frank's wife the DBT skills will increase her ability to recognize his skillful behavior, prompt skillful behavior, and reinforce accordingly.

Skills training, particularly validation skills, are common components of marital interventions. In turn, a stable marital relationship is associated with decreased recidivism (Bogue, 2002).

14. What would be the issues to be addressed in termination? How would termination and relapse prevention be structured?

As mentioned earlier, forensic treatment must target violent recidivism (Hodgins, 2002). Frank's Violence Relapse Plan must be addressed prior to termination. This work is typically completed in group therapy (McCann et al., 2000) but is adaptable to individual format.

In brief, following completion of basic DBT, Frank would develop a relapse plan incorporating data from previously completed behavioral analyses on all violent behavior. Frank would document the following: precipitating events, vulnerability factors, interfering emotions, skills deficits, reinforcers of ineffective behaviors, and punishers of effective behaviors. This document is followed by a solution and repair plan. The solution plan addresses the factors listed above. The repair plan addresses how Frank can correct and overcorrect the consequences of his violence. Please see McCann and colleagues (2000) for details.

15. What do you see as the hoped for mechanisms of change for this patient, in order of relative importance?

Cognitive behavior therapies, including DBT, focus on four primary mechanisms for problem behavior:

1. lack of needed skills,
2. environmental contingencies favor ineffective behavior rather than more adaptive behaviors,
3. emotions interfering with the ability to behave effectively, and
4. cognitions interfere with the ability to behave effectively.

DBT adds to this model by highlighting the role of emotions in driving ineffective behaviors and suggests five deficits that lead to problematic emotion based behavior: (a) inability to regulate physiological responses (e.g., muscle tension and resulting body language, breathing, pounding heart, "tunnel vision"), (b) inability to move attention away from distressing or infuriating cues (e.g., ability to physically turn or walk away from situation, ability to mentally change attention to a new topic vs. ruminating), (c) inability to experience emotions without escalating them (e.g., sadness today means an inevitable future of failures) or blunting or masking them, (d) inability to block mood-dependent, impulsive behaviors, and (e) inability to mobilize behavior in the service of long-term goals.

Thus, in DBT the mechanism of change will be the remediation of these deficits. The order of events generally starts with a combination of a slow but steady increase in knowledge and competence in skillful behaviors (especially in the 5 emotion-deficit areas) facilitated by new environmental contingencies that stop reinforcing ineffective behaviors (e.g., safe alternatives to therapists and family giving in to threatening and blaming behaviors are implemented) and increase reinforcement for the skillful alternatives. Some of the latter are a natural consequence of skillful behavior, but much will be manufactured by the therapist as part of shaping awkward approximations of the behavior into truly skillful means. As this process stabilizes the patient's situation, more exposure and cognitive modification strategies are added to address the problems of interfering emotions and thoughts, respectively.

REFERENCES

Allard, T.J., Wortley, R.K., & Steart, A.L. (2003). Role conflict in community corrections. *Psychology, Crime, & Law, 9*, 279–289.

Andrews, D. A., & Bonta, J. (1998). *The psychology of criminal conduct.* Cincinatti, OH: Anderson Publishing Company.

Berner, A.E., & Warner, G.M. *An introduction to contemporary psychoanalysis.* New York: Jason Aronson.

Berzins, L.G., & Trestman, R.L. (2004). The development and implementation of Dialectical Behavior Therapy in forensic settings. *International Journal of Forensic Mental Health, 3,*

Bogue, B. (2002). *An Evolutionary Model for examining Community Corrections.* Boulder, CO: Justice System Assessment & Training.

Dimeff, L., Rizvi, S. L., Brown, M., & Linehan, M. M. (2000). Dialectical Behavior Therapy for substance abuse: A pilot application to methamphetamine-dependent women with Borderline Personality Disorder. *Cognitive and Behavioral Practice, 7*, 457–468.

Fruzzetti, A.E., & Levensky, E.R. (2000). Dialectical Behavior Therapy for domestic violence: Rationale and procedures. *Cognitive & Behavioral Practice, 7*, 435–446.

Hare, R.D. (2003). *Hare PCL-R technical manual*, (2nd ed.). N. Tonawanda, NY: MHS.

Hodgins, S. (2002). Research priorities in forensic mental health. *International Journal of Forensic Mental Health, 1*, 7–23.

Hodgins, S., & Cote, G. (1993). Major Mental Disorder and Antisocial Personality Disorder: A criminal combination. *Bulletin of the American Academy of Psychiatry & Law, 21*, 155–160.

Hollander E., Allen, A., Lopez, R., Bienstock, C., Grossnan, R., Siever, L., et al. (2001). A preliminary double-blind, placebo-controlled trial of divalproex sodium in cluster B personality disorders. *Journal of Clinical Psychiatry, 62,* 199–203.

Lieb, K., Zanarini, M., Schmahl, C., Linehan, M.M., & Bohus, M. (2004). Borderline Personality Disorder. *Lancet, 364,* 453–461.

Linehan, M. M. (1993a). *Cognitive-behavioral treatment of borderline personality disorder.* NY: Guilford.

Linehan, M. M. (1993b). *Skills training manual for treating borderline personality disorder.* NY: Guilford.

Linehan, M. M. (1997). Validation and psychotherapy. In A. Bohart & L. Greenberg (Eds.), *Empathy reconsidered: New Directions.* Washington, DC: APA.

Linehan, M. M. (Speaker). (2000). *Opposite action: Changing emotions you want to change* (Video Tape). Seattle, WA: Behavioral Tech LLC.

Maslach, C., & Jackson, S.E. (1993). *Maslach burnout inventory.* Palo Alto, CA: Consulting Psychologists Press.

McCann, R.A., & Ball, E.M. (1996, November). *Using Dialectical Behavior Therapy with an inpatient forensic population.* Workshop presented at the first annual meeting of the International Society for the Improvement and Teaching of Dialectical Beahvior Therapy (ISITDBT), New York.

McCann, R.A., Ball, E. M., & Ivanoff, A. (2000). DBT with an inpatient forensic population: The CMHIP model. *Cognitive & Behavioral Practice, 7,* 447–456.

McCann, R.A., Ivanoff, A., Beach, B., & Schmidt, M. (in press). DBT implementation in long-term forensic settings. In A. Dimeff, K. Koerner, & C. Sanderson (Eds.), *Adaptations of DBT.* New York: Guilford.

Miller, A.L., Rathus, J.H., Leigh, E., & Landsman, M. (1996, November). *A pilot study: Dialectical Behavior Therapy adapted for suicidal adolescents.* Poster presented at the first annual meeting of the International Society for the Improvement and Teaching of Dialectical Behavior Therapy (ISITDBT), New York.

Miller, W.R., & Rollnick, S. (2002). *Motivational interviewing.* NY: Guilford.

Patterson, G. R., DeBaryshe, B. D., & Ramsey, E. (1989). A developmental perspective on antisocial behavior. *American Psychologist, 44,* 329–335.

Swann, W. B., Rentfrow, P. J., & Guinn, J. S. (2002). Self-verification: The search for coherence. In M. Leary & J. Tagney (Eds.), *Handbook of self and identity.* New York: Guilford.

Tangney, J. P., & Dearing, R. L. (2002). *Shame and guilt.* New York: Guilford.

Trupin, E. W., Stewart, D.G., Beach, B., & Boesky, L. (in press). Effectiveness of a Dialectical Behavior Therapy program for incarcerated female juvenile offenders. *Child Psychology and Psychiatric Review.*

Waltz, J., Babcock, J. C., Jacobson, N. S., & Gottman, J. M. (2000). Testing a typology of batterer. *Journal of Clinical and Consulting Psychology, 8,* 658–669.

Watson, D.L., & Tharp, R. G. (1977). *Self-directed behavior: Self-modification for personal adjustment* (2nd edition). Monterey, CA: Brooks/Cole.

Wong, S., & Gordon, A. (2000). *Violence Risk Scale.* Saskatchewan, Canada: Regional Psychiatric Center.

Wong, S. & Hare, R. (1998). *Program guidelines for the institutional treatment of violent psychopathic offenders.* Unpublished manuscript.

Zanarini, M., & Frankenburg, F. (2001). Olanzepine treatment of female borderline personality disorder patients: A double blind, placebo controlled pilot study. *Journal of Clinical Psychiatry, 62,* 849–854.

CHAPTER 9

Motivational Interviewing

Joel I. Ginsburg, C.A. Farbring, and L. Forsberg

Authors' Note: The opinions expressed in this chapter are those of the authors and do not necessarily represent the Correctional Service of Canada, the Swedish Prison Service, or the Karolinska Institute. The authors wish to thank Ruth Mann for her helpful comments on an earlier version of this chapter.

I. Treatment Model.

Motivational interviewing (MI; Miller & Rollnick, 2002) originates from the field of alcohol-abuse treatment. It was developed in response to the failure of confrontational approaches to treating individuals who abuse alcohol. While not originally intended to be a treatment per se, MI can produce changes in behaviors such as problem drinking and other substance misuse (Bien, Miller, & Tonigan, 1993; Burke, Arkowitz, & Dunn, 2002; Ginsburg, 2000; Miller, 2000). Motivational interviewing is a client-centered approach that explores and resolves client ambivalence in favor of positive behavior change (Miller & Rollnick). It focuses on building motivation for and fostering a commitment to change. Empirical research supports its use with individuals who abuse alcohol and other substances (Burke, Arkowitz, & Menchola, 2003).

Motivational interviewing addresses motivational struggles in behavior change. Motivation is not conceptualized as a client trait. Instead, motivation is fluid, occurs in an interpersonal context, and is influenced by the interaction of counselor and client. Motivation is not something that is instilled in the client. Instead, intrinsic motivation is evoked from the client. While MI includes techniques to enhance motivation, it is first and foremost a method of communicating with clients (Miller & Rollnick, 2002). There is a "spirit" or "way of being" with the client that is central to the approach. This style of communication facilitates the evocation of natural change processes in the client (Rollnick & Miller, 1995). The spirit of MI is characterized by a part-nership between client and counselor that honors the client's perspective and self-knowledge in an atmosphere that is safe and conducive to change (Miller & Rollnick). The client's freedom to choose whether he/she wishes to change is affirmed. Additionally, the client is viewed as autonomous and possessing the resources and motivation for change.

Brief mention will be given to four guiding principles underlying MI: express empathy, develop discrepancy, roll with resistance, and support self-efficacy (Miller & Rollnick, 2002). First, MI is built on reflective listening that conveys accurate empathy and the counselor's acceptance of the client. Second, change is facilitated by focusing on discrepancies between the client's present behavior and his/her goals and values. Third, resistance to change is not opposed directly. Instead, resistance is acknowledged, new perspectives may be provided, and the client is viewed as a primary source for solutions. Fourth, the counselor's belief in the client's ability to change is as important as the motivating effect of the client's belief in the possibility of change and his/her capacity to change.

Given that MI is a client-centered approach, it might be of concern to counselors working with offenders in light of findings discussed by Gendreau (1996). He noted that nondirective/client-centered interventions have gener-ally been ineffective in reducing offender recidivism. However, while MI is client-centered, it is also directive by focusing on developing discrepancy, resolving ambivalence about change, and using reflective listening to selec-tively reinforce change talk (e.g., a client speaking about the possibility of change.) and decrease resistance to change (Miller & Rollnick, 2002).

Motivational interviewing has been discussed and used in the context of criminal justice populations (Amrod, 1997; Ferguson, 1998; Ginsburg, 2000; Ginsburg, Mann, Rotgers, & Weekes, 2002; Harper & Hardy, 2000; Mann, Ginsburg, & Weekes, 2002; Miller, 1991, Vanderburg, 2002). As with drinkers, confrontation is equally ineffective with offenders. Perhaps offend-ers, like substance abusers in community samples, will respond positively to the gentler and more respectful approach of MI (Miller).

Research has generated principles of classification for effective correc-tional rehabilitation (Andrews, Bonta, & Hoge, 1990). These principles assist counselors in identifying suitable treatment candidates, identifying appropri-ate treatment targets, and intervening in a manner that matches key characteristics of the client to effect behavior change. When viewed in this context, MI is linked to the responsivity principle (Andrews & Bonta, 2003). This principle guides counselors to match their intervention to important client characteristics like readiness to change.

The goal of using MI with offenders is not exclusively related to reducing recidivism, although this would be a welcome outcome. Instead, MI can be used as a pretreatment primer to enhance readiness for existing treatment protocols (Jamieson, Beals, Lalonde, and Associates, 2000). Or, MI can be used adjunctively with other interventions to enhance their potency (Saunders, Wilkinson, & Phillips, 1995). For example, MI integrates well with cognitive-behavioral interventions to form a broader treatment framework (Baer, Kivlahan, & Donovan, 1999; Bien, Miller, & Boroughs, 1993).

Motivational interviewing's focus on client responsibility for change integrates well with the stages of change (Prochaska, DiClemente, & Norcross, 1992). These stages provide information about the client's readiness to change. (In MI, "readiness" is viewed in the context of the importance of change to the client and his/her confidence in his/her ability to change.) The first phase of MI builds motivation for change and assists clients in moving from the pre-contemplation and contemplation stages to the preparation stage. The second phase of MI strengthens commitment to change with clients in the preparation stage. Motivational interviewing can also be used to support self-efficacy in clients who have relapsed (e.g., a parolee who has violated a condition of release).

Research findings from a related motivational intervention are germane to this discussion. Motivational Enhancement Therapy (MET; National Institute on Alcohol Abuse and Alcoholism, 1995) is an adaptation of MI. It includes an assessment battery followed by four individualized treatment sessions. The first two sessions include the client's "significant other." Assessment feedback is provided; then MET builds motivation and consolidates commitment to change.

A large-scale study (Project MATCH) revealed that MET was more effective than Cognitive Behavior Therapy and Twelve Step Facilitation Therapy for clients who present for alcohol-disorders treatment with high anger ratings (Miller & Longabaugh, 2003). The authors suggest that the non-confrontational approach of MET differentially benefits angry clients by diminishing their resistance. Sociopathy, severity of alcohol use, and related psychological problems did not affect response to MET (Project MATCH Research Group, 1997a, 1997b). These findings suggest that MI, as the building block of MET, might have special relevance to offenders given that they frequently present in treatment as angry. Despite findings from earlier research (Kadden et al.,

2001), Project MATCH did not produce any effects when treatments were matched with sociopathy.

Ethical concerns have been raised about using MI with clients who have not expressed a desire to change (Miller, 1994; Rollnick & Morgan, 1995). However, this dilemma might be less problematic when working with offenders. In this case, there is an argument for intervening to reduce the risk of recidivism and thereby contributing to societal protection. Miller and Rollnick (2002) address other ethical considerations including power imbalances faced by parole officers who wish to use MI with their clients.

II. Clinical Skills.

The clinical skills most essential to using MI are reflective listening, responding to change talk, and responding to resistance (Miller & Rollnick, 2002). Reflective listening can be viewed as the "glue" that binds the techniques of MI. It provides the substance of the approach. Motivational interviewing's strong emphasis on using reflective listening makes it client-centered. Reflective listening is used to encourage clients to talk in session and perceive themselves as being understood. Further, it conveys counselor empathy, warmth, and acceptance. Also important is the counselor's ability to remain neutral and nonjudgmental. Miller & Rollnick recommend a particular emphasis on using reflective listening during the early stage of MI.

Apart from being client-centered, MI is also directive by focusing on resolving ambivalence to facilitate change, often in a particular direction (Miller & Rollnick, 2002). For example, a counselor working with a substance-abusing client might use MI to facilitate behavior change towards less substance use. The counselor selectively reflects "change talk" or client statements that move toward change. Amrhein (2003) discerns four underlying dimensions of change talk: problem recognition (cognitive dimension), need (emotional dimension), ability, and desire. The mere wish to change is insufficient for successful behavior change. Commitment language ("do-language") from the client is also needed for behavior change. Change talk, specifically strength of commitment language, is associated with decreased use of drugs (Amrhein, Miller, Yahne, Palmer, & Fulcher, 2003). Thus, client commitment language is an important "compass" for assisting the counselor in guiding the client towards change.

When clients express disadvantages of their present behavior, speak of the advantages of change, voice optimism about change, or discuss intention to change, they are emitting change talk. The counselor responds to the change talk by elaborating, reflecting, summarizing, and affirming by using reflective listening. By reflecting change talk the counselor gives the client an opportunity to hear his/her own statements a second time. On the other hand, resistance or client verbalizations that move away from change are not reinforced so they will diminish. Thus, the counselor responds differentially to the client's verbalizations. The simultaneous occurrence of change talk and resistance illustrates ambivalence.

Instead of arguing for one side of ambivalence (e.g., change) only to be met by the client arguing for the other side of ambivalence (not changing), MI guides counselors to acknowledge ambivalence as understandable and a natural part of behavior change (Miller & Rollnick, 2002). If resistance is encountered, then instead of opposing it directly, the counselor "rolls with it." Rolling with resistance often requires the counselor to use reflective listening skillfully to convey to the client that he/she has listened and understood. Such a reflection might reduce resistance and it may be followed by additional techniques. For example, resistance can be reframed. The client is invited to take a new perspective and momentum towards change can be re-established.

Some counselors view resistance as a client trait. In MI, resistance is viewed as a product of the interpersonal interaction between counselor and client. Resistance signals the counselor that he/she and the client are not working together. It is a cue for the counselor to change his/her behavior (Miller & Rollnick, 2002). Thus, resistance is a counselor problem, not a client problem.

Motivational interviewing provides the counselor with specific means of responding to resistance. These range from simple reflections to more amplified ones, and more complex reflections like double-sided reflections which reflect both sides of the client's ambivalence. Reflection is not the only way of responding to resistance. Other responses include shifting the client's focus away from the "barrier," reframing the client's resistance, emphasizing the client's freedom of choice and autonomy, and at the extreme, siding with the client and defending his/her option to not change.

III. Questions.

1. Primary and secondary goals. (Long-term and short-term goals.)

Clinically speaking, Frank is a delicate person to work with. How do you work with an individual who is perceived by almost everyone as being truly unsympathetic? By concentrating on the individual's experience, social learning history, frame of reference, and values, it is often possible to understand him better, which is an explicit goal of MI. Goals are elicited from the client, but nonetheless the counselor works with behavior change as a goal. The primary therapeutic goal could be reducing Frank's alcohol abuse. Given the events that led to Frank's referral, this could impact on the secondary goal: reducing Frank's parole violations and more generally limiting his violations of the criminal laws. Frank ultimately decides which goals, if any, will be chosen. Other options could include decreasing threatening behavior, increasing use of social skills, and sharing more of his thoughts with significant others (e.g., his wife). A short-term goal for the counselor is to establish rapport with Frank in a safe counseling environment so that Frank does not feel threatened.

2. Further information.

Additional information from recent contact (if any) between Frank and his brother would be interesting. This might answer the following questions: Has Frank offered any remarks about his brother recently? Has Frank's opinion of his brother changed? Is there any affection expressed between them? The counselor should focus on examples of pro-social thoughts and behaviors that could assist in achieving treatment goals.

3. Conceptualization of personality, behavior, affective state, cognitions.

Case conceptualization is not part of the MI approach; however, the following comments are provided. Frank is likely to be hypersensitive to criticism and suggestions about behavior change. This reaction to feedback might lead to resistance (e.g., aggressive behavior), thus making it difficult to establish rapport. Frank perceives others (especially those whom he is mandated to see) as potential threats; therefore he seeks control over them and the ensuing situations. It is important for Frank to perceive himself as being strong physically and psychologically. Possessing power is important to Frank.

The counselor could take the stance that there are many problems in Frank's life that could be addressed and then elect to work from a directive stance. But this does not mean that the counselor will tell Frank what is best for him or what he needs to do. Motivational interviewing strives to empower the client, so that he/she exercises control over his life and related choices and decisions.

4. Pitfalls and difficulties; sources of difficulties.

Potential pitfalls include directing Frank's attention prematurely towards problems and behavior change. Suggestions implying criticism or need for improvement could engender resistance, thereby creating obstacles to establishing rapport. Ultimately this can lead to treatment failure (Amrhein, Knupsky, et al., 2003). Client responses, including resistance to counselor behavior, provide the counselor with immediate feedback on which he/she can gauge the success of his/her interactions with the client (Miller, Benefield, & Tonigan, 1993). Counselor behavior can directly affect the degree of client resistance, which, in turn, is highly predictive of negative treatment outcome (Amrhein et al., 2003; Miller et al., 1993; Miller & Sovereign, 1989; Moyers, 2003; Patterson & Forgatch, 1985).

Miller and Rollnick (2002) list various traps to avoid in MI, including: asking too many questions, portraying oneself as "the expert," labeling the client's behavior, and blaming the client.

Finally, evidence suggests that MI can be difficult to learn and practice effectively (Miller & Mount, 2001; Miller, Yahne, Moyers, Martinez, & Pirritano, in press). Therefore, the counselor's level of expertise could act as a potential pitfall. Moyers (2003) notes that if counselors attend to client change talk and resistance, and tailor their behavior accordingly, then they will gain proficiency in using MI. However, counselor proficiency is also associated with training and receiving supervised feedback from taped MI sessions (Amrhein, Miller, Yahne, Knupsky, & Hochstein, 2003).

5. Expected level of success. Immediate and long-term result?

Our hope is that Frank will be open to exploring and learning about his behavior, contemplating and committing to behavior change, and perhaps even engaging in behavior change as a result of the MI. Perhaps Frank's alcohol abuse will decrease. He might show additional adaptation by abiding by his parole conditions and breaking fewer laws. Other long-term behavior change might result from the generalization of positive reinforcement that Frank might receive from simply giving change a try. According to research and theory cited in this chapter, prognosis can be predicted by examining the prevalence of resistance behavior and the intensity of change talk during counseling.

6. Duration of counseling.

We recommend starting with five, hour-long, weekly semi-structured MI sessions. Follow-up will be provided as an option to Frank. We will use a "driver's guide" through MI (Farbring & Berge, 2003), a protocol employed within the Swedish criminal justice system. A description of the sessions follows.

Session 1. The counselor creates an environment in which Frank perceives that he is understood as a person, not just as a client. This is best achieved by using reflective listening. The counselor remains cognizant that Frank is a mandated client. Links are drawn between Frank's present situation and his lifestyle. The counselor attempts to elicit Frank's thoughts and feelings about his current situation. Certain words like "problems" are not used by the counselor because Frank will likely interpret them as an insult and then respond with resistance. Frank will most likely consider change if it will help him to increase control over his life and if it is congruent with his values. The counselor will support change that is pro-social in its direction. Assuming that Frank will change only if there are clear benefits for him, it is important for the counselor to be aware of potential sources of reinforcement (e.g., personal empowerment, restoring social balance with his wife, reducing the need for parole supervision).

The concept of change is introduced by the counselor in a calm and neutral manner. For example, changes related to eating, physical activity, weight management, smoking, and so forth are discussed as engaging many people daily. This serves as an introduction to stimulating Frank's curiosity about changes that he might pursue. Examples are elicited that focus on changes that are most important to Frank (e.g., getting his wife back, reducing problems with parole staff and other authorities, following an occupation with less potential for legal difficulties).

Session 2. The counselor continues to develop discrepancy between Frank's present antisocial lifestyle and a more pro-social lifestyle in which he has fewer problems with authorities and more control over his life. The counselor attempts to elicit specific problem recognition (without ever using the expression) and emotional distress from Frank regarding his present situation compared to what might be a better alternative (Saunders, Wilkinson, & Allsop, 1991). It is important to allow Frank to explore and elaborate in his own words the positive and negative consequences of his current lifestyle and the negative and positive consequences of an alternate lifestyle. To start the "motor of change" in MI, the counselor attempts to evoke distress from Frank about his present situation. A mere intellectual understanding of the "problem" is insufficient as a catalyst for change.

Session 3. The counselor continues to develop discrepancy by focusing on emotional elements. Miller & Rollnick (2002) recently introduced the concept of "behavior gap." The counselor must be careful not to make the gap between the present behavior and the desired behavior too wide. If problem recognition and subjective distress are increased to levels at which Frank feels overwhelmed by the degree of change that is required, then his self-efficacy will diminish and he will not view change as possible. However, there is reason to believe that Frank, like certain other clients, generally overestimates his perceived resources in almost any area (Demmel & Rist, 2002). Nevertheless, it is important that the counselor does not create a behavior gap that is too great for the client to bridge.

Session 4. Here the focus is on Frank's values and his network of important associates. Frank's value system is probably very simple, comprised of values that serve him best in the short-term. The counselor communicates acceptance of Frank as a person and respect for his values even if the counselor disagrees with these values. Important gains can be realized when the counselor helps Frank see that his values comprise an important component of his unique personality and provide a system that helps guide his life (Rokeach, 1973). If there are discrepancies between Frank's values and his lifestyle, then his views on these discrepancies are elicited with a view of creating emotional tension. The counselor might focus on alcohol abuse and antisocial behavior but the final decision remains with Frank regarding the behaviors and change (if any) that he wishes to address.

Frank is probably less dependent on his social network than other individuals are on their respective networks. Nevertheless this topic needs to be examined. Frank has acquaintances, some of whom are afraid of him while others admire him. He makes good use of social skills when he wants to and often he can be charming and persuasive. The following questions will guide part of the session: What types of individuals appeal to Frank? What are the advantages to having a network of reliable people whom he trusts? Does Frank cultivate these types of friends? What, if anything, is "not so good" about Frank's social network? How could his relationship with his wife improve?

Session 5. The counselor will summarize progress to date, including examples of change talk, and then ask Frank what he'd like to do next. Normally the aim of this session is to define behavior(s) to be changed and make a concrete change plan. However, it is possible that this agenda might seem provocative to Frank; therefore a "softer" way of proceeding might be more appropriate. If Frank is not yet ready to proceed towards developing a behavior change plan, then the counselor can continue to build motivation for change. For example, the counselor can summon Frank to explore the future by asking him to imagine and describe how he would like his life to be in a few years. The process continues by asking Frank to describe the steps that are necessary to get there. The session ends by thanking Frank for his cooperation and asking if he would like to continue examining his situation.

7. Specific techniques

Motivational interviewing provides counselors with techniques for listening and exploring that emphasize understanding the client. These techniques include open questions, affirming, reflective listening, and summaries (OARS). The techniques are a means of following the principles of

MI which were discussed earlier. Further, MI offers a "compass" (Amrhein et al., 2003a,b) which directs the counselor towards eliciting and reinforcing change talk from the client as well as reducing resistance.

Recall that by attending to client change talk and resistance, the counselor can gauge his/her effectiveness in working with the client. With Frank, the counselor recognizes that his participation in counseling is not entirely voluntary; therefore, respecting the MI approach, it will be especially important to avoid using persuasion or providing advice without solicitation or Frank's permission. Despite efforts to minimize the likelihood of resistance, if it is encountered then the principle of rolling with it will be followed. The following sample transcript of interactions with Frank will illustrate features of the MI approach.

> *Counselor (C): Frank, I realize that this might be an unusual situation for you and that the decision to come here was not entirely yours. If you are willing, I would appreciate it if you would tell me a bit about how things are going for you at the moment. I would also like to know how I might be helpful to you during our time together. Is this agreeable with you?* The opening dialog is very important. It will not be surprising if we encounter resistance from Frank due to his situation and the nature of his referral. There is a risk that too much elaboration on his resistance will create difficulty for further discussion about his situation. The counselor's aim is to recognize and reflect resistance and to change focus by placing resistance in the "parking lot."

> *Frank (F): Well, you're right. I don't want to be here and I really don't like this situation at all. I have no idea what we are going to talk about or how you can be helpful to me. I am not used to getting any help from authorities or other people. I usually take care of myself.* Frank's somewhat hostile tone is not unexpected. Recognizing Frank's resistance, the counselor will be cautious in his/her approach and try not to stir up any more resistance.

> *C: Being independent and having control over your life is important to you.* This reflection invites Frank to elaborate on what has gone wrong, given that he has lost some control over his present situation. This will guide us towards an important principle of MI: developing discrepancy between Frank's current situation and where he would like to be. Emotional discomfort arising from this discrepancy is described as the *"motor of change"* (Miller & Rollnick, 2002; Saunders et al., 1995). A potential pitfall is moving too quickly to the detriment of establishing rapport and a safe environment for Frank to self-disclose. After Frank's confirmation that he wants to control his life and destiny, the counselor continues:

> *C: Frank, aside from having had control over your life, your successful military career suggests that you have had significant responsibility over*

others. By **affirming** one of Frank's strengths, the counselor strives to make the atmosphere less threatening. Further, this action communicates to Frank that he is "seen" as an individual and not as a generic client. Increased comfort leads to increased self-disclosure. In MI, the client should be doing most of the talking, not the counselor. To this end, **open questions** are used judiciously to stimulate responses that are more elaborate than "yes/no."

C: Frank, how do you feel about your life at the moment? This simple open question invites Frank to focus on what is important at the moment. Hopefully he will discuss what is bothering him.

F: I don't like being harassed by all these authorities and you people.

C: I can understand that this is really frustrating for you. Can you tell me a little bit about what caused this? The counselor's goal is for Frank to discuss his drinking and disorderly conduct. Open questions permit Frank to hear himself talk about his situation, whereas if the counselor tells Frank what is wrong with his situation then there is a significant risk of engendering resistance. Open questions provide an opportunity for Frank to recognize what could be a better situation for him. In this case, the counselor follows up with open questions aimed at eliciting change talk. Below, Frank discusses the events that led to his arrest:

F: I was having a beer in a bar, just relaxing and talking. Then some guys started making a lot of noise and pulling pranks. Everyone thought that they were real goofs so I told them to leave. They didn't, so I helped them leave. Somebody must have called the cops but they arrested me instead of them!

C: You took action and made things happen. When this happens you can be really persuasive and make people do as you want. How does your history as an officer come into play? The counselor aims to have Frank elaborate on his impulse to get into fights and to recognize a possible pattern of violent behavior. After exploring this pattern, the counselor will ask Frank to discuss the "good things" and the "not so good things" about fighting. Questions are interspersed among copious examples of **reflective listening** to avoid the "question-answer trap," a situation well-known to clients who have been interrogated by police, social welfare agencies, and other authorities.

Reflective listening provides the client with a "receipt" indicating that the counselor has heard and understands what has been said. It communicates to the speaker (Frank) that the listener (Counselor) is interested in Frank's story and what it means to him. The counselor carefully chooses material to reflect, thereby allowing the client to hear his words once again. This process provides the client with strong social and contextual reinforcement. Reflections can remain within the limits of what has been said but sometimes the counselor will focus on the emotion connected to the client's words.

Miller & Rollnick (2002) introduced *"continuing the paragraph,"* a more advanced form of reflective listening. This technique goes beyond what the client has said. It is a hypothesis about what could or would be said if the client thought a few steps ahead about change. This technique is preferable to asking an open question because it does not require an answer and hopefully it will guide the client toward change.

F: *I think all this is blown out of proportion. I don t have a drinking problem. All I did was what anyone would have done if he had the guts to stand up for himself.*

C: *You are a man with a strong sense of integrity.* This reflection is also an affirmation. This reflection is directive because it changes Frank's focus from complaining about the situation and allows the counselor to guide exploration of behavior change in the following exchange with Frank.

F: *Yes, it seems that I have to defend myself against you people and authorities all the time.* Frank could probably elaborate for a long time on this topic. Here we abbreviate this conversation to illustrate how things can progress.

C: *Still, situations like this come up and this is not at all what you want.* Hopefully Frank will agree and present an opportunity for exploration.

F: *Right, this really sucks!*

C: *So, how could things be different? Is there anything you could do to get the authorities off your back?* The goal of using this open question it to "pull" for change talk from Frank. The counselor is directing the conversation towards change.

F: *I really don't know. I just know that I need to do something. I just can't take this harassment anymore.*

C: *This is all too much for you and you're looking for ways to avoid this in the future.* This reflection underscores Frank's discomfort and it is oriented toward change talk. Frank admits that he needs to do something, so the counselor has "struck gold." As we will see soon, reflective listening encourages Frank to continue speaking by elaborating on his situation.

F: *It's hell!* Communicating in the style of MI with Frank is completely opposite to the way in which he relates and talks to others. It will probably seem strange to Frank but hopefully it will convey genuine respect, which might be equally foreign to Frank.

Some of our trainees have asked whether reflective listening conveys to the client that the counselor supports the client's problem behavior. Thus, can the client distinguish between support for him/her as an individual (reflective listening) and support for his/her problem behavior? Our clinical experience indicates that clients do not confuse our support for them as individuals with support for their problem behavior.

Another technique used in MI is providing the client with **summaries.** These can be used to reinforce positive statements about change that the client has uttered. The client hears what he/she has said a second time. Even though the counselor is vocalizing the summary, he/she uses words that the client has used to enhance the salience and meaningfulness of the summary for the client. The summary should be accurate; however, the counselor can add an interpretation to the summary. This can assist the client in understanding the meaning of what he/she has said.

Summaries can be used any time that the counselor wishes to illuminate something that is important for the client. Summaries are also commonly used at the conclusion of a counseling session. Summaries often follow with a question to the client: *"Did I get this right or is there anything that you want to add?"* An example follows:

C: Frank, you had strong feelings about being harassed by the authorities and you don't think that your drinking was any of their business. Negative content is described in the past tense at the beginning of the summary. Positive content follows and it is expressed in the present tense. Using the present tense underscores that the positive content is important "right here and right now."

C: You also believe that there are things that you can do to prevent situations like this from happening. Having developed discrepancy and by using the open question that follows, the counselor aims to elicit change talk from Frank. Frank will be influenced to a large degree by what he hears himself say. He will be influenced very little, if at all, by what others (including the counselor) tell him to do.

C: So Frank, what can you can do about this? There are many possible paths to reach this point and, once there, the counselor "remains" with the client so that more change talk can be elicited. Directing the client towards and listening for change talk is like digging for gold; you are not leaving the gold until all of it has been extracted (Barth, Prescott, & Börtveit, 1999).

First, the counselor focuses on developing discrepancy by juxtaposing Frank's value of being in control with his present situation.

C: So now that you do not have full control of your life, what kind of feelings does that cause inside you? How would you feel if this situation was to continue for years? By inviting Frank to look to the future and envision no change, the counselor attempts to magnify Frank's discomfort and encourage him to elaborate on it.

F: I'll never accept that. That is not going to happen.

C: You will not tolerate that. So what is the next step? The counselor uses reflective listening and follows with a key question to elicit change talk. At this point it is imperative that the counselor continue to avoid giving advice.

F: I suppose I could make myself less interesting to them so that they would stop harassing me in the future.

C: In what way? The counselor is "digging for gold."

F: Well, alcohol is one area. Not that I have any problem with it. But I suppose I could cut down anyway.

The counselor will continue to "dig in this gold vein" until Frank has specified the commitment to change that he is willing to undertake. Later, the counselor might try to develop discrepancy between other deeply held values and Frank's present situation. For now, there is one sensitive area for the counselor's focus.

C: Now you are living alone, at least temporarily, although we don't know if it will be permanent. How do you feel about that? This is a sensitive topic for Frank because he has tried to persuade his wife to return to him. The open question aims at increasing Frank's discomfort.

F: Well, I'll get her back. I know I can. Until just recently we had a good life together.

C: Your wife is very important to you. What can you do to help restore her confidence in you? A reflection is used to mirror an important relationship for Frank. Bandura (1997) emphasizes the relationship between self-efficacy and behavior change. Nothing indicates that Frank believes he is lacking in self-efficacy. As stated earlier, he likely has an inflated opinion about his capabilities in general. Instead of focusing on Frank's skills, the counselor shifts focus to what Frank thinks he must *do* to change his wife's perception of him.

F: I guess she does not like to worry about my legal situation but she is reading too much into what has happened. Frank acknowledges his wife's worry but then he minimizes it.

C: She is concerned about you and worrying about your life together. How can you increase her comfort with you? A reflection is followed by a key question aimed at eliciting change talk.

F: I don't know. Maybe I could tell her more about my job.

C: Telling her more about your legal means of earning income to make her feel safe. The counselor is reflecting on the edge of what Frank has said by continuing the paragraph.

F: Yeah, something like that.

C: Your military success has provided you with the discipline needed to make changes. Once you make a decision, you follow through on it. Affirmation is used to reinforce Frank's strengths. The counselor will target a behavior that Frank will be willing to change.

F: Yes, I know I can do anything I set my mind to.

C: And what are you thinking of right now that would help you reach the kind of situation you want to have?

F: Well, I don't know really; getting a stable job would probably help.

C: You wouldn't need to handle situations where legality is put in doubt.

F: That's right.

C: So what kind of job would be acceptable to you?

F: As things are right now, I guess I could take just about any job to get out of this situation. The conversation continues and the counselor tries to elicit more change talk from Frank, preferably in *"do language"* by continuing to explore and develop discrepancy. It is best to concentrate on a few areas during the five sessions instead of attempting to cover Frank's complete life situation.

8. Cautions to be observed. Expected resistance.

There are no special cautions to be observed when using MI with Frank. As illustrated in the previous section, resistance can be expected given the nature of Frank's referral and his circumstances. Some other examples of resistance follow:

F: You are just like all the other "Nine to Five" people that I have met. All you are doing is collecting a paycheck and using your power. In this situation, the counselor takes a step back and reflects the feeling underlying Frank's resistance. The purpose is to focus on rapport and leave the change work for later.

C: I can see that you really don't want to be here. You are probably pretty upset. I'm wondering whether I might have said or done something that is bothering you?

F: You are right about me not wanting to be here but it doesn't have to do with anything that you did or said.

C: Frank, if there is ever anything that I say or do that upsets you then please tell me, because I don't want to be causing you any more difficulty than you are already experiencing. Okay?

F: Okay.

C: I'd like to help you so that you don't have to go to different places and meet with different people whom you really don't want to see. Given that you and I will be working together, perhaps you can tell me how you would like to use our time together?

Supporting the client's autonomy, freedom of choice, and responsibility for change can be an effective means of rolling with resistance.

C: Frank, what you want to do with your life is completely up to you. I can only give you support if you want it. I cannot and will not try to persuade you to do anything that you don't want to do. Also, the information that you might take from our sessions is for your use or you might decide not to use it. It's up to you. After resistance has subsided, the counselor will use a "compass bearing" in the direction of change (Amrhein et al., 2003a,b). This is the overarching goal of our sessions with Frank.

9. What would be avoided.

There are not any areas that we would avoid with this client. However, Frank is the ultimate decision-maker regarding topics for discussion and behavior to be changed. The counselor will aim to follow the "driver's guide" (Farbring & Berge, 2003) described earlier, while remaining cognizant that the best "guide" is often the words that the client has just said. The "driver's guide" provides a route to follow through the MI landscape. The counselor will navigate cautiously through the sessions in an attempt to minimize resistance and other bumps in the journey.

10. Medication.

We do not see any need to refer Frank to a psychiatrist. An absence of psychotropic medication should not have any effect on the efficacy of MI. If Frank wishes to try a pharmaceutical to assist him in changing his drinking behavior then this will be discussed during counseling and his wish will be supported.

11. Strengths of Frank.

Frank is a keen observer of others. He is adept at determining individuals' reinforcers and he can use social skills when needed. Frank is independent and a problem solver. He is capable of following his own path but he can also adapt to environments that include others.

12. Limits, boundaries to be addressed with Frank.

The counselor's use of the "driver's guide" combined with the accompanying principles and techniques should keep Frank within the boundaries of behavior change and prevent him from getting sidetracked.

The counselor will be careful not to cross Frank's boundaries. For example, Frank might decide that discussing his brother is not negotiable.

Frank might try to assert his control and test the counselor's limits by asking personal questions. This can be addressed with reflective listening and rolling with resistance. If necessary, Frank will be told that this is not a topic for exploration. For example, Frank might inquire about the counselor's drinking habits. The counselor could ask Frank why this is important to him and then answer the question briefly including a statement about the topic's relevance (e.g., minimal relevance to practicing MI with Frank.).

If Frank violates the counselor's personal space by sitting in close proximity or touching him/her, then the counselor will gently alert Frank to this behavior, discuss it with him in a neutral and respectful manner, and if necessary set some "ground rules" for counseling.

13. Involvement of significant others. Homework.

The participation of significant others is not part of the MI framework. However, as discussed earlier, MET is an offshoot of MI and it provides for the participation of significant others early in the intervention.

Similarly, the use of homework is not a component of MI; however, if Frank requests to do work out-of-session then this could be examined.

14. Issues to be addressed in termination. Relapse prevention.

The counselor will reinforce that all of the information learned and the interaction that took place in the sessions is material for Frank to use or not use, depending on his wishes. If Frank desires additional counseling then this could be discussed. Additional counseling would continue building motivation to change and strengthening commitment to change. Recall that MI is not a method for instructing clients on how to change.

While MI can be used in the context of relapse, relapse prevention is not part of MI. The counselor and Frank could discuss different paths that Frank could follow for the future, including the possible consequence of the various directions that Frank could take.

15. Hoped for mechanisms of change in order of relative importance.

Motivational interviewing is influenced by various psychological theories, including self-perception theory (Bem, 1967), which speaks of an important mechanism of change. This theory tells us that individuals learn what they hear themselves say. Therefore, using reflective listening to reinforce change talk is a mechanism of change.

Motivational interviewing provides a style of communication and a "way of being" with the client that fosters natural change processes that reside within the individual (Miller & Rollnick, 2002; Sobell & Sobell, 1993).

Developing discrepancy between the client's present behavior and his/her goals and important values is another mechanism of change. It is important for the discrepancy to have an emotional dimension for the client.

Self-efficacy or the availability of a means to change and the client's perception of his/her ability to succeed in behavior change is predictive of change and another example of a mechanism of change (Bandura, 1997).

REFERENCES

Amrhein, P. C. (2003). *A training manual for coding client commitment language* (version 1.0). Upper Montclair, NJ: Department of Psychology, Montclair State University.

Amrhein, P. C., Miller, W. R., Yahne, C. E., Knupsky, A., & Hochstein, D. (2003a). Strength of commitment language during motivational interviewing increases with therapist training. *International Conference on Treatment of Addictive Behaviors—10* poster.

Amrhein, P. C., Miller, W. R., Yahne, C. E., Palmer, M., & Fulcher, L. (2003). Client commitment language during motivational interviewing predicts drug use outcomes. *Journal of Consulting and Clinical Psychology*, 71(5), 862–878.

Amrod, J. (1997). The effect of motivational enhancement therapy and coping skills training on the self-efficacy and motivation of incarcerated male alcohol abusers (Doctoral dissertation, University of Missouri, 1997). *Dissertation Abstracts International*, 57(9-B), 5904.

Andrews, D. A., & Bonta, J. (2003). *The psychology of criminal conduct* (3rd ed.). New York: Anderson.

Andrews, D. A., Bonta, J., & Hoge, R. D. (1990). Classification for effective rehabilitation. Rediscovering psychology. *Criminal Justice and Behavior*, 17(1), 19–52.

Baer, J. S., Kivlahan, D. R., & Donovan, D. M. (1999). Integrating skills training and motivational therapies: Implications for the treatment of substance dependence. *Journal of Substance Abuse Treatment*, 17(1–2), 15–23.

Bandura, A. (1997). *Self Efficacy. The exercise of control.* New York: W.H. Freeman.

Barth, T., Prescott, P., & Börtveit, T. (1999). Endringsfokusert rådgivning. Endringsfokusert rådgivning. Gyldendal Akademisk.

Bem, D. J. (1967). Self-perception: An alternative interpretation of cognitive dissonance phenomena. *Psychological Review*, 74, 183–200.

Bien, T. H., Miller, W. R., & Boroughs, J. M. (1993). Motivational interviewing with alcoholic outpatients. *Behavioural and Cognitive Psychotherapy, 21*, 347–356.

Bien, T. H., Miller, W. R., & Tonigan, J. S. (1993). Brief interventions for alcohol problems: A review. *Addiction, 88*, 315–335.

Burke B., Arkowitz, H., & Dunn, C. (2002). The efficacy of motivational interviewing and its adaptations. In W. R. Miller, & S. Rollnick (Eds.), *Motivational interviewing: Preparing people for change* (pp. 217–250). New York: Guilford Press.

Burke, B., Arkowitz, H., & Menchola, M. (2003). The efficacy of motivational interviewing: A meta-analysis of controlled clinical trials. *Journal of Consulting and Clinical Psychology*, 71(5), 843–861.

Demmel, R., & Rist, F. (2002). Infaltionäre Selvstwirksamkeitserwartungen alkoholabhängiger Patienten. MINUET, May.

Farbring, C.Å., & Berge, P. (2003) Beteende—Samtal—Förändring. Fem semis-trukturerade motiverande samtal (pp. 1—125). Kriminalvårdsstyrelsen, Nor-rköping.

Ferguson, R. T. (1998). Motivational interviewing with less motivated driving under the influence of alcohol second offenders with an exploration of the processes related to change. (Doctoral dissertation, University of Wyoming, 1998). *Dissertation Abstracts International*, 59(1-B), 0415.

Gendreau, P. (1996). Offender rehabilitation. What we know and what needs to be done. *Criminal Justice and Behavior, 23*(1), 144–161.

Ginsburg, J. I. D. (2000). *Using motivational interviewing to enhance treatment readiness in offenders with symptoms of alcohol dependence*. Unpublished doctoral dissertation, Carleton University, Ottawa, Ontario, Canada.

Ginsburg, J. I. D., Mann, R. E., Rotgers, F., & Weekes, J. R. (2002). Using motivational interviewing with criminal justice populations. In W. R. Miller & S. Rollnick (Eds.), *Motivational interviewing: Preparing people for change* (pp. 333–346). New York: Guilford Press.

Harper, R., & Hardy, S. (2000). An evaluation of motivational interviewing as a method of intervention with clients in a probation setting. *British Journal of Social Work, 30*, 393–400.

Jamieson, Beals, Lalonde, & Associates, Inc. (2000). *Motivational Enhancement Treatment (MET) manual. Theoretical foundation and structured curriculum. Individual and group sessions*. Developed for the State of Maine, Department of Mental Health, Mental Retardation and Substance Abuse Services, Office of Substance Abuse. Ottawa, Toronto, Canada: Author.

Kadden, R., Litt, M., Cooney, N., Donovan, D., Stout, R., & Longabaugh, R. (2001). Sociopathy as a client-treatment matching variable. In R. Longabaugh, P. Wirtz, & F. Del Boca (Eds.), *Project Match hypotheses: Results and causal chain analyses*. Bethesda, MD: National Institute on Alcohol Abuse and Alcoholism.

Mann, R. E., Ginsburg, J. I. D., & Weekes, J. (2002). Motivational interviewing with offenders. In M. McMurran (Ed.), *Motivating offenders to change: A guide to enhancing engagement in therapy* (pp. 87–102). Chichester: John Wiley.

Miller, W. R. (1991). Emergent treatment concepts and techniques. *Annual Review of Addictions Research and Treatment, 2*, 283–295.

Miller, W. R. (1994). Motivational interviewing: III. On the ethics of motivational intervention. *Behavioural and Cognitive Psychotherapy, 22*, 111–123.

Miller, W. R. (2000). Rediscovering fire: Small interventions, large effects. *Psychology of Addictive Behaviors, 14*, 6–18.

Miller W.R. (2002, November). A streetcar named desire. *Minuet*. Volume 9, pp 1–4.

Miller, W. R., Benefield, G., & Tonigan, S. (1993). Enhancing motivation for change in problem drinking: A controlled comparison of two therapist styles. *Journal of Consulting and Clinical Psychology, 61*, 455–461.

Miller, W. R., & Longabaugh, R. (2003). Summary and conclusions. In T. Babor, & F. Del Boca (Eds.), *Treatment matching in alcoholism*. Cambridge, MA: Cambridge University Press.

Miller, W. R., & Mount, K. (2001) A small study of training in motivational interviewing: Does one workshop change clinician and client behavior? *Behavioral and Cognitive Psychotherapy, 29*, 657–671.

Miller, W. R., & Rollnick, S. (Eds.). (2002). *Motivational interviewing. Preparing people for change* (2nd ed.). New York: Guilford Press.

Miller, W. R., & Sovereign, G. (1989). The check-up: A model for early intervention in addictive behaviors. In T. Löberg, W. R. Miller, P. Nathan, & A. Marlatt (Eds.), *Addictive behaviors, prevention and early intervention* (pp. 219–229). Amsterdam: Swets & Zeitlinger.

Miller, W. R., Yahne, C. E., Moyers, T., Martinez, J., & Pirritano, M. (in press). A randomized trial of methods to help clinicians learn motivational interviewing. *Journal of Consulting and Clinical Psychology*.

Moyers, T. (2003) *What should we be teaching? Using process analyses to guide training*. Tenth international conference on treatment of addictive behaviors. Presentation. Heidelberg, Germany.

National Institute on Alcohol Abuse and Alcoholism, U.S. Department of Health and Human Services. (1995). *Motivational enhancement therapy manual: A clinical research guide for therapists treating individuals with alcohol abuse and dependence* (Project MATCH Monograph Series, NIH Publication No. 24–3723). Rockville, MD: Author.

Patterson, G., & Forgatch, M. (1985). Therapist behavior as a determinant for client noncompliance: A paradox for the behavior modifier. *Journal of Consulting and Clinical Psychology, 53*, 846–851.

Prochaska, J. O., DiClemente, C. C., & Norcross, J. C. (1992). In search of how people change. Applications to addictive behaviors. *American Psychologist, 47*(9), 1102–1114.

Project MATCH Research Group. (1997a). Matching alcoholism treatments to client heterogeneity: Project MATCH posttreatment drinking outcomes. *Journal of Studies on Alcohol, 58*, 7–29.

Project MATCH Research Group. (1997b). Project MATCH secondary a priori hypotheses. *Addiction, 92*(12), 1671–1698.

Rokeach, M. (1973). *The nature of human values*. New York: Free Press.

Rollnick, S., & Miller, W. R. (1995). What is motivational interviewing? *Behavioural and Cognitive Psychotherapy, 23*, 325–334.

Rollnick, S., & Morgan, M. (1995). Motivational interviewing: Increasing readiness for change. In A. M. Washton (Ed.), *Psychotherapy and substance abuse. A practitioner's handbook* (pp. 179–191). New York: Guilford Press.

Saunders, B., Wilkinson, C., & Allsop, S. (1991). Motivational intervention with heroin users attending a methadone clinic. In W. R. Miller & S. Rollnick (Eds.),

Motivational interviewing. Preparing people to change addictive behavior (pp. 279–292). New York: Guilford Press.

Saunders, B., Wilkinson, C., & Phillips, M. (1995). The impact of a brief motivational intervention with opiate users attending a methadone programme. *Addiction, 90,* 415–424.

Sobell, M. B., & Sobell, L. C. (1993). *Problem drinkers.* New York: Guilford Press.

Vanderburg, S. A. (2002). *Motivational interviewing as a precursor to a substance abuse program for offenders.* Unpublished doctoral dissertation, Carleton University, Ottawa, Ontario, Canada.

CHAPTER 10

Integrating Psychotherapy and Medication

Sharon Morgillo Freeman and John M. Rathbun

Discussion of biological treatments for antisocial personality disorder (ASPD) occasions much frustration among scientists and clinicians. This disorder includes problems such as irritability, deceit, illegal behaviors with little or no remorse, hostility, aggressiveness, impulsivity, and very often manipulative charm. Not only is there controversy regarding treatment options, but opposed camps have arisen; some hold that there is no known pharmacologic treatment for ASPD, others that there is treatment but science has not discovered it yet, or that some aspects of the syndrome are treatable while others are not (Dinwiddie, 1994, 1996; Hirose, 2001; Stringer & Josef, 1983; Walker, Thomas & Allen, 2003).

To cloud the picture even further, the *Diagnostic and Statistical Manual of Mental Disorders—Fourth Edition Text Revision* (DSM) (American Psychiatric Association, 2000) represents an attempt to impose categorical thinking on phenomena that are inherently multi-dimensional (Tuinier & Verhoeven, 1995). The diagnosis of ASPD is a prime example of difficulties that arise when attempting to apply DSM-IV-TR criteria to the typical patient. Application of DSM criteria for ASPD includes the near certainty that the same person will also meet, or have met, criteria for one or more additional psychiatric diagnoses (Swanson, Bland, & Newman, 1994). Our own experience finds that illnesses commonly comorbid with ASPD include substance misuse disorders, mood disorders, and various disruptive behavior disorders such as attention-deficit hyperactivity disorder, oppositional-defiant disorder, and conduct disorder. Researchers have also pointed out that ASPD comorbid with other disorders, such as substance misuse, predicts a poor prognostic picture for psychotherapeutic intervention (Woody, McLellan, Luborsky, & O'Brien, 1985). The common factor in each of these overlapping categories is a failure to control impulses destructive to the peace and safety of others.

People with impulse-control problems are often profoundly self-destructive. The pain to their victims and close associates is palpable. But the word "patient" may not apply to such persons until they choose to accept that role. Engendering and nurturing a therapeutic alliance with people whose behavior is manipulative, impulsive, and dangerous is a challenge for any clinician.

The possibility of genetic transmission of certain behaviors, such as impulsiveness and destructiveness (Coccaro, Bergeman, & Kavoussi, 1997), implies that certain behavioral traits may be a product of brain structure. This implication has fueled the search for biological interventions that would adjust brain function to reduce a person's potential for acting on destructive impulses. It is against this background of cultural and conceptual confusion that we attempt to describe biological approaches to the treatment of Antisocial Personality Disorder. We will focus on those symptoms most amenable to pharmacologic intervention: aggressive and impulsive behaviors.

DIAGNOSTIC CHALLENGES

Our journey begins with the descriptive confusion in the DSM criteria regarding ASPD. In an effort to improve reliability, the authors constructed criteria that include psychopaths but also a larger population of non-psychopathic offenders. The distinction is important to a discussion of treatment possibilities, since the literature distinguishes two types of aggression that occur in persons with ASPD: impulsive aggression and planned aggression. The latter is more characteristic of psychopathology, and there is no known medical treatment of planned aggression in criminal behavior.

On the other hand, impulsive aggression has been the subject of much study in human and animal populations, and there are some relevant medical treatments. We recommend caution on this point, since it is possible to see both types of aggression in the same person, and many aggressive acts cannot be definitely characterized. In considering what sort of treatment to recommend to a person with ASPD, it is important to take an extensive history, including from collateral sources, and make your best judgment about what sort of aggression predominates.

A third variety of aggression that must be ruled out is aggression from medical illness. Substance abuse (common in ASPD), delirium, dementia, infection, head injury, and endocrine/metabolic problems are the main medical considerations in the differential diagnosis of aggression. Major psychiatric diagnoses on Axis I of the DSM may also explain increased aggression (such as bipolar disorder, substance misuse, and delirium). Psychotic disorders, including mood disorders of psychotic intensity, are particularly apt to give rise to aggression. For these reasons, a careful medical and psychiatric history, physical examination, and indicated laboratory testing are mandatory in the evaluation of aggression. We will provide a brief discussion of the specific biological inferences as we discuss specific symptomatology for ASPD.

PATHOPHYSIOLOGY OF AGGRESSION AND IMPULSIVITY

There is a virtually infinite array of things that can go wrong with the development and maintenance of the human brain, beginning with genetic factors and progressing through antenatal, perinatal, neonatal, childhood, and adult occurrences. Physical traumas that result in frontal lobe lesions, such as anoxia, malnutrition, infection, irradiation, endocrine/metabolic disturbances, and poisonings are among the most common non-genetic causes of cerebral imperfections that may lead to impulsive and/or aggressive behaviors (Murad, 1999). Simpson and colleagues suggest that traumatic brain injury (TBI) was a significant etiological factor (6.5%) with sexually aberrant behaviors over alcohol as a factor (2.3%) in a population of adult sex offenders (Simpson, Blaszczynski, & Hodgkinson, 1999). In addition, Slaughter, Fann, and Ehde (2003) reported that 87% of inmates in a county jail population had a TBI during their lifetime, 36.2% in the prior year. Similar results are reported by Tateno and colleagues in a population of patients with a history of TBI; 33.7% exhibited aggressive behavior post-injury (Tateno, A., Jorge, R. E., & Robinson, R.G., 2003). Children who have experienced a traumatic brain injury are more likely to exhibit higher levels of loneliness, maladaptive behavior, and aggressive/antisocial behaviors. These children, upon reaching adult age, may be considered ASPD-impaired if the history of TBI and the sequela are not known, given that the behaviors would be seen as pervasive and lifelong.

Aggression is an extremely complex, unsettled, and rapidly-evolving area of neurobiology. A full discussion of recent research findings is beyond the scope of this chapter, so the reader is encouraged to consult a basic neurobiology text such as Shepherd (1994).

In brief, emotional behavior (analogous to Freud's *id* energy) is generated by primitive structures that lie deep in the brain, specifically the *basal ganglia*. Human ability to refrain from acting on our emotional impulses is primarily attributed to the function of more recently developed parts of the brain that control rational analysis and social judgment. The human brain differs from animal brains especially in the size and dominance of *our cerebral cortex,* the part that gives us our characteristically oversized head. In psychoanalytic terms, we could consider this outer part of the brain to be the organ of the *ego.* In fact, there has been some progress in the evaluation of brain structure and function in persons with impulse control, aggression, and chronic disinhibition. Raine and colleagues (1994) found evidence of hypoactivity in the prefrontal structures of persons convicted of murder who exhibited symptoms similar to ASPD. Other researchers point to bilateral lesions of the orbitofrontal cortex and medial face of the frontal lobe (Grafman et al., 1996; Murad, 1999) as possible explanations for antisocial behaviors.

Impulsive behaviors reflect inadequate cortical dominance in the stimulus-response paradigm. Such persons are perceived as *childish* or immature by their peers, because young children have limited cortical development and tend to express their impulses freely, while mature adults are characterized by considerable behavioral inhibition in the service of good social relations.

Investigations of human psychophysiology are retarded by practical and ethical considerations, funding gaps, and the lack of a satisfactory animal model for the human brain. We do have considerable indirect evidence that the basic physiology of human aggression and impulsivity is in many ways similar to what we have found in animal brains. Animal research into the neurobiology of aggression has revealed a number of chemical substances that serve as modulators of activity in the basal ganglia and cerebral cortex (Horn, Dolan, Elliott, Deakin, & Woodruff, 2003). These substances include serotonin (Panksepp, Yue, Drerup, & Huber, 2003), dopamine (Cardinal, Winstanley, Robbins, & Everitt, 2004), norepinephrine, acetylcholine, glutamate, γ-aminobutyric acid, and testosterone among others (Whybrow, 1994). To make matters more complicated, the brain contains several types of receptor sites for each of these substances, so a single substance can produce direct inhibition of some structures while simultaneously stimulating activity elsewhere. Even more complexity is added by the existence of numerous interconnections among brain cells and structures, allowing for a plethora of indirect influences and negative feedback loops.

Numerous exogenous chemicals can modulate brain neurochemistry. These include naturally occurring substances present in our environment as well as synthetic chemicals, legal and otherwise. Such neuroactive chemicals give us much indirect information about the underlying pathophysiology of impulsive behavior. The general theory that applies is that cortical enhancers and basal ganglia suppressors support good impulse control, while opposite effects in the brain are associated with increased incidence of impulsive aggression (Murad, 1999).

For these reasons, a thorough physical and neurological evaluation with laboratory examinations as indicated by special circumstances is mandatory in the evaluation of impulsive aggression. Further, major psychiatric disturbances on Axis I of the DSM may explain aggressive behavior; such problems must be evaluated before an accurate diagnosis of Axis II problems becomes feasible, and definitive treatment of personality problems is usually facilitated by resolution of acute problems on Axis I.

A thorough discussion of medical and psychiatric evaluation protocols needed to rule out major problems on Axis I and Axis III of the DSM is beyond the scope of this article.

IMPULSIVITY AND AGGRESSION

It is important to understand that impulsiveness is not just bad judgment. The emerging consensus among medical researchers is that impulsiveness is better understood as NO judgment. The research suggests a prefrontal screening process that takes less than half a second, before the person has time to become conscious of the relevant stimuli (Barratt, 1993).

The normal outcome of such screening is a "referral" to cortical centers that are specialized for conscious consideration of the situation and a rational decision about how to respond (Davidson, Putnam, & Larson, 2000). Percepts that match paradigms of imminent serious threat, such as SNAKE HERE NOW, are shunted to central urgent threat-response centers before conscious awareness of the threat develops. This emergency response mode is evidenced by changes in autonomic nervous system function which are detectable sooner than the cortical arousal patterns associated with threat analysis (Bechara, Damasio, Tranel, & Damasio, 1997).

Some persons appear to have a lowered threshold for the irrational threat-response mode to be activated. These persons do not always manifest other psychopathology, and may show genuine remorse after an aggressive action. Their behavior may meet the DSM criteria for ASPD, and therefore be an appropriate target for psychopharmacologic intervention.

We are indebted to Swann (2003) for his synthesis of available data on impulsive aggression. His analysis indicates a delicate balance between excitatory and inhibitory influences on aggressive behavior. In general, the neurotransmitter serotonin tends to inhibit aggression, while dopamine tends to release aggression (Van Praag, Asnis, & Kahn,1990). Other neurotransmitters are also relevant insofar as they affect the general arousal level: glutamate increases arousal whereas gamma-amino butyric acid (GABA) reduces it. The effects of some mood-altering chemicals on aggression may be mediated by glutamate and GABA, while severe Axis I psychiatric disturbance is associated with abnormalities in serotonin and dopamine levels. Abuse of stimulants, especially cocaine, could produce aggressive effects through increasing both dopamine and norepinephrine levels.

Nicotine has been found to have potent anti-aggressive effects, possibly because of its influence on serotonin (Seth, Cheeta, & Tucci, 2002). Nicotine withdrawal is associated with increased aggression that can be moderated by use of nicotine gum (Cherek, Bennett, & Grabowski, 1991). Testosterone levels have been found to be abnormally high in persons who exhibit aggressive behaviors (Gerra, Zaimovic, & Avanzini, 1997), and the use of androgenic steroids, such as in cases of body building, is associated with variable increases in aggression (Pope, Kouri, & Hudson, 2000). The complexity of the interacting systems described above suggests multiple methods might be useful in the management of impulsive aggression. Certainly the elimination of toxins such as alcohol, androgens, and stimulants is mandatory.

THE CASE OF FRANK

The case of "Frank" that leads off this discussion presents a person who meets DSM criteria for ASPD. Given the limited information, it is not clear whether he has impulsive aggression absent alcohol intoxication. His alcohol abuse certainly requires further investigation to determine whether he meets DSM criteria for alcohol dependence. Cocaine abuse would not be a surprising finding in such a person, and could explain some of his adult symptoms. Given the possibilities of substance-induced aggressive behavior, a urine drug screen should be conducted early in Frank's evaluation. It is also possible that Frank may have a bipolar or unipolar depression. His moodiness, which includes expansive moods alternating with dour, brooding, surly spells, requires that the clinician evaluate for disorders comorbid with his Axis II disorders.

Frank probably met DSM criteria for conduct disorder and for attention deficit hyperactivity disorder (ADHD) in childhood. A more interesting question, from the psychopharmacologist's point of view, regards the tonic (hyperthymia) or intermittent (hypomania) presence of excessive energy and expansive mood. These states can be confused with ADHD when they occur in childhood, and could explain many of his adult traits of high energy, charm, irritability, impulsiveness, flamboyance, risk-prone lifestyle, and expansive ego. One instance of psychological testing is insufficient to rule out a major mood disorder, since most mood disorders follow an intermittent, fluctuating, or cyclical course. An accurate diagnosis of mood disorders often depends on serial observations (Hantouche et al, 1998). Additional testing would be helpful, in addition to collateral history obtained from Frank's family and significant others.

A thorough assessment of risk and dangerousness is the main priority for any team managing such patients. The most salient index of the severity of the ASPD is the degree of dangerousness. These patients are at elevated risk for death from impulse-related behavior that could produce an immediate catastrophe (such as when Frank jumps off a cliff) or longer-term disaster (such as HIV/AIDS acquired from unprotected sexual encounters).

TREATMENT CHALLENGES

A general aim of treatment is to improve the patient's motivation to comply with societal laws and expectations in regards to sexual behavior, substance use, occupational productivity, and respect for the privacy and property of others. Getting Frank to assume the role of "patient" will be among the most challenging aspects of his treatment. He does not see his behavior as a problem for him, and he does not care how it affects others. In this frame of mind, he will not easily be led to stop poisoning his brain with alcohol and other substances, nor will he readily agree to let a doctor medicate him. Therefore it will be imperative to explore reasons for Frank to change his behavior. Many times this may be as simple as saying, "Let's find a way for you to be less bothered by nosy parole officers!" or "We may be able to find a way to get your wife to stop her complaining, so you can enjoy your freedom." What we actually propose here is a partnership to get Frank to cease obnoxious behaviors so his wife will have fewer reasons to complain.

Clinical experience suggests that persons with ASPD become treatable mainly when they are trapped in a situation of powerlessness and are experiencing considerable pain. This may occur because of legal prosecution, or when the consequences of their behavior result in significant depression or threatened loss of a valued relationship. Much the same logic applies to substance abusers and persons with hyperthymia. Frank's presenting situation in the vignette may give the therapist sufficient initial leverage, but the work will likely be long, hard, and a little dangerous.

If Frank is severely hyperthymic, he may not be amenable to most forms of psychotherapy because the neurochemical output of his basal ganglia would often override cortical control. In other words, the impulsivity may win out in most cases.

MEDICATION OPTIONS

Most studies of pharmacologic treatment of personality disorders have been conducted in persons with diagnoses in cluster B, and especially in antisocial and borderline personality disorders. Partial positive results have been obtained using various classes of drugs for dealing with aggression and impulsive behaviors, including lithium, beta-blockers, carbamazepine, valproate, antipsychotic drugs, and SSRIs (Swann, 2003).

Lithium salts

Numerous published studies going back to the dawn of modern psychopharmacology have shown the benefits of lithium salts in a variety of contexts. Lithium was the first specific treatment for mania, and has since proved effective in hypomania, treatment-refractory depression, and intermittent explosive disorder (Grof, & Grof, 1990). Although its safe use requires considerable expertise, it is commonly effective against impulsive aggression in doses that are well-tolerated by most patients. Lithium raises synaptic serotonin levels modestly, and has more important effects on intracellular second-messenger systems. Lithium's effects are usually apparent within 2 weeks when it is given aggressively.

Serotonergic agents

Among the most commonly prescribed substances in modern psychiatry are the selective serotonin reuptake inhibitor (SSRI) antidepressants such as fluoxetine (Prozac), paroxetine (Paxil), sertraline (Zoloft), citalopram (Celexa), and escitalopram (Lexapro). These drugs are easy to use and relatively safe even when a patient deliberately overdoses. Other serotonergic agents exist but are not so commonly used in American medical practice. Coccaro and Kavoussi (1997) showed that impulsive aggression responds to SSRI treatment. Forty subjects with personality disorders and histories of impulsive aggression received either fluoxetine 20 to 60 mg daily or placebo for 12 weeks. Fluoxetine reduced the incidence of overt aggression and irritability by about 67%. Re-analysis by the same authors suggest that SSRIs may be most effective in moderately aggressive patients (Lee & Coccaro, 2004) whose serotonergic system may be less impaired than that of highly aggressive patients (Coccaro, Kavoussi, & Hauger, 1997). The beneficial effects of SSRIs are typically delayed at least 2 weeks, and agitation can be temporarily exacerbated by these agents.

Anticonvulsants

Impulsively aggressive subjects who do not respond to an SSRI may respond to an anticonvulsant (Kavoussi, & Coccaro, 1998). An anti-aggressive response in impulsive aggressive persons has been reported for carbamazepine (Cowdry & Gardner, 1988), diphenylhydantoin (Barratt, Stanford, Felthous, & Kent, 1997), and valproic acid (Lindenmayer & Kotsaftis, 2000). Anticonvulsants can become effective within minutes when a loading dose is given under close medical supervision.

Antipsychotic drugs

Drugs that have been approved for treatment of psychosis fall into two broad categories. The older agents (chlorpromazine, perphenazine, fluphenazine, haloperidol, and others) are dramatically effective against agitation and aggression within minutes, and haloperidol can be given intravenously when seconds count. They are not the first choice in non-emergency treatment of aggression, however; their uncomfortable side-effects make them an unpopular option for most patients and doctors. In chronic use, they may cause a disfiguring movement disorder called *tardive dyskinesia* that can become permanent. In the best hands, the older antipsychotics commonly sap a patient's vitality, producing the dreaded "zombie" effect.

A new generation of antischizophrenic medications has come to the fore in the past 15 years. These currently include clozapine, olanzapine, risperidone, quetiapine, ziprasidone, and aripiprazole, with more in the pipeline. These agents are known to reduce aggressive behavior in psychotic illness without the muscular side-effects typical of older antipsychotics; their use in impulsive aggression, absent psychosis, is based on inference and a paucity of rigorous clinical studies. The newer antipsychotics do not work as fast as the older ones, but their overall effect on mood and social function is considered much superior by psychopharmacologists generally.

Beta-Blockers

Propranolol and other agents developed for the treatment of hypertension and tachycardia have been shown to be effective in a variety of contexts where anxiety and aggression are the target symptoms (Haspel, 1995). Because this agent is indicated for hypertension it can cause faintness and occasionally depression, and is therefore not considered a first-line agent by most practitioners.

Dopaminergic agents

Substances that increase dopamine activity in the brain, such as amphetamines and methylphenidate, would not ordinarily seem a logical choice in the treatment of aggression, given that dopamine excess generally facilitates aggression in animals and humans. Many young persons and some adults may actually benefit from dopamine's alerting effects when defective impulse inhibition is a consequence of cortical under-arousal. Such individuals commonly meet DSM criteria for attention deficit disorder (ADD) that is often comorbid with conduct disorder or ASPD. In such cases, stimulant treatment may restore cortical dominance and actually reduce aggression (Connor, Glatt, & Lopez, 2002).

Sedative-hypnotics

Benzodiazepine tranquilizers are sometimes used parenterally for acute treatment of aggression, often lorazepam in combination with haloperidol. They work in seconds when given intravenously. Lorazepam can also be given intramuscularly, where it works in a few minutes. These compounds have serious disadvantages in chronic use: habituation, dependence, and tachyphylaxis are common; paradoxical aggression is not rare. Other types of sedatives are rarely used due to their potential to cause respiratory depression.

Sex steroids

Anti-androgen compounds have shown some benefit in demented and brain-injured patients. Advantages include the availability of long-acting injectable preparations that enhance compliance. Estrogen has been tried but well-designed studies are lacking. These sex steroids have a long list of disagreeable and dangerous side-effects, making them unattractive in most cases.

OPTIONS FOR FRANK

As mentioned above, removal of toxins from Frank's brain would be an initial priority from the psychopharmacologist's point of view. A complete medical evaluation is needed, both to rule out other medical causes of his symptoms and to bring to his attention any evidence of physical damage caused by his substance misuse, fighting, and high-risk lifestyle. Involvement of a physician or advanced practice nurse at this stage is important because a person with medical-psychiatric training can more convincingly present the medical evidence and answer his questions. Use of a high-status professional may also be helpful because of Frank's narcissism.

People with ASPD are prone to addiction and drug-seeking behaviors, and may also be prone to sell their medications rather than take them. All controlled substances, therefore, would be relatively contraindicated. Should a *bona fide* need for such a medication arise, the quantity should be carefully controlled. Any frequency of "lost" prescriptions would be highly suspicious. Among the medications we could recommend, if Frank becomes amenable, would be lithium carbonate. This underused mineral has the potential to deflate hyperthymia, inhibit impulsive aggression, and even reduce the attractiveness of alcohol. We have had difficulty convincing some patients that lithium is a useful option because they believe that it is used only in severely chronically mentally disabled persons, and that it causes a lot of dangerous and distressing side-effects. With sensitive management and careful monitoring, we find lithium to be well-tolerated and very effective in the milder forms of moodiness that are much more common than psychotic mania. Additionally, the ready availability of serum lithium levels facilitates monitoring of patient compliance in cases like Frank's.

Topiramate is another medication to consider; it has been shown to reduce alcohol abuse (Johnson et al., 2003) and might also have benefits in impulsive aggression. If Frank were overweight, it might be useful to point out that topiramate can cause significant appetite suppression and weight loss, hoping to gain his cooperation through an appeal to his narcissism. Hollander, Tracy, and Swann (2003) reported greater reduction in impulsivity and aggression when persons with DSM cluster B personality disorders were treated with divalproex versus placebo. Interestingly, divalproex was no more effective than placebo in the reduction of impulsivity and aggression in subjects who did not have a diagnosis of cluster B personality disorder.

Antipsychotic Medications

Rocca, Marchiaro, Cocuzza, and Bogetto (2003) found significant reduction in aggression scores with risperidone in persons with borderline personality disorder. The results were based on Aggression Questionnaire scores. This amelioration was coupled with an overall improvement in depressive symptoms and an increase in energy and global functioning. A review of the literature by Markovitz (2004) regarding the use of atypical antipsychotics in both schizotypal personality disorder and antisocial personality disorder from 2000 through 2003 documented a pattern of encouraging outcome reports.

We think that the alternative psychopharmacologic options mentioned above would be less helpful than lithium or topiramate in a case like Frank's. Serotonergic agents could aggravate his hyperthymia, and he probably wouldn't like the side-effects; we would expect him to be particularly intolerant of sexual side-effects. The dopamine blockade caused by typical antipsychotics would give him a very disagreeable loss of physical vigor, and the threat of persistent tardive dyskinesia would not please him at all. GABA-ergic medications such as minor tranquilizers are generally habit-forming and he would probably abuse them; they could also cause paradoxical aggression through a mechanism similar to that of alcohol. Such measures as chemical castration would be unlikely to win his informed consent. Anticonvulsants other than topiramate have side-effects, such as weight gain, sluggishness, and tremor, which would most likely lead to psychological rejection. Beta-blockers would not help his hyperthymia, and stimulants are contraindicated in most aggressive adults because they increase dopamine levels.

OPTIMISTIC PROGNOSTIC FACTORS

Because Frank is intelligent, he would respond best to a therapist who is willing to engage his desire to become "expert" on most topics. Experiments testing hypothetical outcomes of behavior changes might entice him. Additionally, he could possibly be challenged to investigate his physiologic responses to medications with the prospect of publishing his "case study."

Frank's wife has indicated that she is invested in Frank's recovery and remains connected to him. Her willingness to support his recovery should be explored. The possibility of a pharmacologic intervention may encourage her to remain supportive, given her forgiving nature; that might provide Frank some motivation for adhering to a medication treatment plan. In most cases, successful pharmacotherapy of Frank's disorder would require a life-long commitment. He would likely need frequent doctor visits at the outset and continued medical supervision indefinitely.

SUMMARY

Pharmacologic treatment of ASPD is an uncertain undertaking. The core features of sociopathy are not productive targets for currently available medications. Impulsive aggression is the most important target for medical treatment in ASPD. Lithium salts, various anticonvulsants, some beta-blockers, antipsychotics, serotonergic antidepressants, anti-androgen agents, and in some cases even stimulants may benefit impulsive aggression. These agents should be prescribed and monitored by a thoroughly-trained psychopharmacologist. An appropriate medical evaluation should be performed to rule out health problems that can cause or exacerbate impulsive aggression, or complicate its treatment.

REFERENCES

American Psychiatric Association. (2000). *Diagnostic and Statistical Manual of Mental Disorders, Fourth Edition–Text Revision.* Author: Washington, DC.

Barratt, E.S. (1993). The use of anticonvulsants in aggression and violence. *Psychopharmacology Bulletin, 29*(1), 75–81.

Barratt, E.S., Stanford, M.S., Felthous, A.R., & Kent, T.A. (1997). The effects of phenytoin on impulsive and premeditated aggression: A controlled study. *Journal of Clinical Psychopharmacology, 17,* 341–349.

Bechara, A., Damasio, H., Tranel, D., & Damasio, A. (1997). Deciding advantageously before knowing the advantageous strategy. *Science, 275,* 1293–1295.

Cherek, D.R., Bennett, R., & Grabowski, J. (1991). Human aggressive responding during acute tobacco abstinence: Effects of nicotine and placebo gum. *Psychopharmacology* (Berlin), *104,* 317–322.

Coccaro, E.F., Bergeman, C.S., & Kavoussi, R.J. (1997). Heritability of aggression and irritability: A twin study of the Buss-Durkee Aggression Scales in adult male subjects. *Biological Psychiatry, 41,* 273–284.

Coccaro, E.F., Kavoussi, R.J. (1997). Fluoxetine and impulsive aggressive behavior in personality disordered subjects. *Archives of General Psychiatry, 54,* 1081–1088.

Coccaro, E.F., Kavoussi, R.J., Hauger, R.L. (1997). Serotonin function and antiaggressive responses to fluoxetine: A pilot study. *Biological Psychiatry, 42,* 546–252.

Connor, D., Glatt, S., & Lopez, I. (2002). Psychopharmacology and aggression, 1: A meta-analysis of stimulant effects on overt/covert aggression-related behaviors in ADHD. *Journal of the American Academy of Child and Adolescent Psychiatry, 41,* 253–261.

Cowdry, R.W., & Gardner, D.L. (1988). Pharmacotherapy of borderline personality disorder: Alprazolam, carbamazepine, trifluroperazine, and tranylcypromine. *Archives of General Psychiatry, 45,* 111–119.

Davidson, R.J., Putnam, K.M., & Larson, C.L.(2000). Dysfunction in the neural circuitry of emotion regulation—a possible prelude to violence. *Science, 289*(5479), 591–594.

Dinwiddie, S.H. (1994). Psychiatric genetics and forensic psychiatry: A review. *Bulletin of the Academy of Psychiatry and Law, 22*(3), 327–342

Dinwiddie, S.H. (1996). Genetics, antisocial personality disorder, and criminal responsibility. *Bulletin of the Academy of Psychiatry and Law, 24*(1), 95–108.

Gerra, G., Zaimovic, A., & Avanzini, P. (1997). Neurotransmitter-neuroendocrine responses to experimentally induced aggression in humans: Influence of personality variable. *Psychiatry Research, 66*, 33–43.

Grafman, J., Schwab, K., Warden, D., Pridgen, A., Brown, H.R,. & Salazar, A.M. (1996). Frontal lobe injuries, violence and aggression: A report of the Vietnam Head Injury Study. *Neurology, 46*(5), 1231–1238.

Grof, P., & Grof, E. (1990). Varieties of lithium benefit. *Progressive Neuropsychopharmacology and Biology in Psychiatry, 14*, 689–696.

Hantouche, E., Akiskal, H., Lancernon, S., Allilaire, J., Sechter, D., Azorin, J., et al. (1998). Systematic Clinical Methodology for validating bipolar II disorder: Data in mid-stream from a French national multisite study (EPIDEP). *Journal of Affective Disorder, 50*, 163–173.

Haspel, T. (1995). Beta-blockers in the treatment of aggression. *Harvard Review of Psychiatry, 2*, 274–281.

Hirose, S. (2001). Effective treatment of aggression and impulsivity in antisocial personality disorder with risperidone. *Psychiatry & Clinical Neuroscience, 55*(2), 161–162.

Hollander, E., Tracy, K.A., & Swann, A.C. (2003). Divalproex sodium is superior to placebo for impulsive aggression in Cluster B personality disorders. *Neuropsychopharmacology, 28*, 1186–1197.

Horn, N.R., Dolan, M., Elliott, R., Deakin, J.F., & Woodruff, P.W. (2003). Response inhibition and impulsivity: an fMRI study. *Neuropsychologia, 41*, 1959–1966.

Johnson, B., Ait-Daoud, N., Bowden, C., DiClemente, C., Roache, J., Lawson, K., et al. (2003). Oral topiramate for treatment of alcohol dependence: A randomized controlled trial. *Lancet, 361*, 1677–1685.

Kavoussi, R.J., & Coccaro, E.F. (1998). Divalproex sodium for impulsive aggressive behavior in patients with personality disorder. *Journal of Clinical Psychiatry, 59*, 676–680.

Lee, R., & Coccaro, E.F. (2004) *Treatment of aggression: Serotonergic agents*. In E.F. Coccaro (Ed.), *Aggression: Assessment and treatment*. New York: Marcel Dekker.

Lindenmayer, J., & Kotsaftis, A. (2000). Use of sodium valproate in violent and aggressive behaviors: A critical review. *Journal of Clinical Psychiatry, 61*, 123–128.

Markovitz, P.J. (2004). Recent trends in the pharmacotherapy of personality disorders. *Journal of Personality Disorders, 18*(1), 90–101.

Mattes, J.A. (2000). Comparative effectiveness of carbamazepine and propranolol for rage outbursts. *Journal of Clinical Neuroscience, 2*, 159–164.

Murad, A. (1999). Orbitofrontal syndrome in psychiatry. *Encephale, 25*(6), 634–637.

Panksepp, J.B., Yue, Z., Drerup, C., & Huber, R. (2003). Amine neurochemistry and aggression in crayfish. *Microscopy Research and Technique, 60,* 360–368.

Pope, H., Jr., Kouri, E., & Hudson, J. (2000). Effects of supraphysiologic doses of testosterone on mood and aggression in normal men: A randomized controlled trial. *Archives of General Psychiatry, 57,* 133–140.

Raine, A., Buchsbaum, M.S., Stanley, J., Lottenberg, S., Abel, L., & Stoddard, J. (1994). Selective reductions in prefrontal glucose metabolism in murderers. *Biological Psychiatry, 36*(6), 365–373.

Rocca, P., Marchiaro, L., Cocuzza, E., & Bogetto, F. (2003). Treatment of borderline personality disorder with risperidone. *Current Psychiatry Reports, 5*(3), 175–176.

Seth, P., Cheeta, S., & Tucci, S. (2002). Nicotinic-serotonergic interactions in brain and behaviour. *Pharmacological Biochemical Behavior, 71,* 795–805.

Shepherd, G.M. (1994). Neurobiology, 3rd. ed. New York: Oxford University Press.

Simpson, G., Blaszczynski, A., & Hodgkinson, A. (1999). Sex offending as a psychosocial sequela of traumatic brain injury. *Journal of Head and Trauma Rehabilitation, 14*(6), 567–580.

Slaughter, B., Fann, J.R., & Ehde, D. (2003). Traumatic brain injury in a county jail population: Prevalence, neuropsychological functioning and psychiatric disorders. *Brain Injury, 17*(9), 731–741.

Soltis, R., Cook, J., & Gregg, A. (2000). Interaction of GABA and excitatory amino acids in the basolateral amygdala: Role in cardiovascular regulation. *Journal of Neurological Science, 17,* 9367–9374.

Stringer, A.Y., & Josef, N.C. (1983). Methylphenidate in the treatment of aggression in two patients with antisocial personality disorder. *American Journal of Psychiatry, 140*(10), 1365–1366.

Swann, A.C. (2003). Neuroreceptor mechanisms of aggression and its treatment. *Journal of Clinical Psychiatry, 64*(Suppl. 4), 26–35.

Swanson, M.C., Bland, R.C., & Newman, S.C. (1994). Epidemiology of psychiatric disorders in Edmonton. Antisocial Personality Disorders. *Acta Psychiatric Scandanavia, 376*(Suppl.), 63–70.

Tateno, A., Jorge, R.E., & Robinson, R.G. (2003). Clinical correlates of aggressive behavior after traumatic brain injury. *Journal of Neuropsychiatry & Clinical Neuroscience, 15*(2), 155–160.

Tuinier, S., & Verhoeven, W. (1995). Dimensional classification and behavioral pharmacology of personality disorders; A review and hypothesis. *European Neuropsychopharmacology, 5,* 135–146.

Van Praag, H., Asnis, G., & Kahn, R. (1990). Monoamines and abnormal behavior: A multi-aminergic perspective. *British Journal of Psychiatry, 157,* 723–734.

Walker, C., Thomas, J., & Allen, T.S. (2003). Treating impulsivity, irritability, and aggression of antisocial personality disorder with quetiapine. *International Journal of Offender Therapy and Comparative Criminology, 47*(5), 556–567.

Whybrow, P.C. (1994). The therapeutic use of triiodothyronine and high dose thyroxine in psychiatric disorder. *Acta Medican Austriaca, 21,* 47–52.

Whybrow, P. (1994). Neuroendocrinolgy. In Frazer, Molinoff & Winokur, (Eds.), *Biological basis of brain function and disease* (pp. 145–162). New York: Raven Press.

Zimmerman, M., Mattia, J., Younken, S., & Torres, M. (1998). The prevalence of DSM-IV impulse control disorders in psychiatric outpatients [Abstract 265]. Annual meeting of the American Psychiatric Association, Washington, DC.

CHAPTER 11

Antisocial Personality Disorder

Summary and Conclusions

Frederick Rotgers

In this final chapter we will attempt to summarize and synthesize the lessons put forward by the authors of our chapters. The case of Frank has been analyzed from eight different perspectives, with each author or authors taking a unique perspective on how to best approach helping Frank become a more productive and satisfied person. Despite the variability in the perspectives, there are a number of common themes that seem to run throughout the chapters. An overarching conclusion from these chapters is that recent thinking and technical advances in treatment generally seem to have reduced the strength of the discouragement that therapists have historically felt in working with patients like Frank. Thus, these chapters present a reason to hope that, for many patients suffering from Antisocial Personality Disorder (APD), treatment can and will be successful in helping them to live more adaptive lives.

Nonetheless, our authors are also far from willing to advance their approaches as a "cure" for patients with APD, at least not in anything approaching the relatively short treatments currently in vogue. Only Benveniste is willing to offer the possibility that Frank may become free of the symptoms that led to his diagnosis of APD in the first place, but that only after a course of treatment that would last 5–10 years. Rather, the overall thrust of the chapters, even the chapter by Freeman and Rathbun on pharmacological approaches, seems to be toward helping Frank manage the more flamboyant and problematic aspects of his behavior, cognitions, and emotions, rather than dramatically changing them.

To organize our summary we will fall back on the same questions we asked our chapter authors. After describing and summarizing the various Treatment Models and Treatment Skills each author considers essential to working with patients like Frank, we will attempt to delineate the similarities and differences among the approaches presented through an examination of the answers to the 15 basic questions the authors addressed. We then offer our own summary and synthesis of these ideas.

The one exception to this approach will be with respect to Freeman and Rathbun's chapter on pharmacological approaches. This chapter, by virtue of the very different scientific and conceptual foundations of pharmacotherapy and psychotherapy, doesn't fit well into the type of analysis we will apply to the other chapters. Rather, we have presented this chapter so the reader can learn about current thinking in the pharmacological intervention with patients with APD, and understand more clearly how medications can be an important adjunct in working with many of these patients. Given these considerations, we omit Freeman and Rathbun's chapter from much of the discussion that follows, except for the answers to the clinical question regarding medication that all chapter authors addressed.

Before we begin, it is important for us to clarify that what follows is our particular view of the chapters. As with any other endeavor, we bring our own training, background, and experiences into the summarizing of these chapters. As a result, we may give short shrift to some aspects of the authors' views, while emphasizing others that, while less important to the authors, seem more so to us. If we misrepresent a particular view in any way, we apologize in advance. We also invite the reader to develop his/her own summary and synthesis of the material presented here, realizing that it may very well differ from ours.

I. Treatment Models.

The treatment models discussed fall along a range from unabashedly psychodynamic to eclectic to unabashedly behavioral, with one approach based in Rogerian concepts. However, only Maniacci, Freeman and Eig, McCann and colleagues, and Ginsburg and colleagues adhere to more or less "pure" models in which the concepts used are largely the result of the work of a single school of therapy.

Benveniste and Maniacci fall toward the psychodynamic end of the range of models. Benveniste focuses almost exclusively on psychodynamic factors, using an approach largely derived from object relations theory but also incorporating ideas from relational psychoanalysis, attachment theory, trauma theory, and at one point in treatment, more behavioral approaches.

Maniacci operates from an Adlerian perspective that, while clearly psychodynamic in its emphasis, focuses less on internal factors than does the more traditional approach of Benveniste. Adlerians view patients in the context of community and the patient's maladaptive behaviors as being due, in part, to psychodynamic factors that prevent adequate integration of personal strengths into a behavior pattern that meshes with the community in which the patient lives. The emphasis here is on altering the functions of the patient's behaviors, often by harnessing strengths to ends different from the ones to which the patients uses them upon entering treatment (e.g., shifting the goal of social perceptiveness from exploitation to establishing a better connection with others in the patient's community).

Dorr's approach, while more technically eclectic than either Benveniste's or Maniacci's, relies on the biosocial learning model developed by Theodore Millon (Millon & Davis, 1996) for its conceptual underpinnings. While maintaining a psychodynamic focus, Dorr also uses concepts derived from biological views of APD (e.g., that some aspects of this disorder may be hereditary or temperament based), as well as incorporating concepts from learning theory at strategic points in treatment. In a sense Dorr bridges the psychodynamic and behavioral models.

Walters's Lifestyle approach is also an eclectic one, incorporating notions from existential therapy, cognitive-behavioral therapy, and evolutionary biology into an approach that aims at changing criminal behavior and criminogenic thinking.

The models followed by Freeman and Eig and by McCann and her colleagues are decidedly non-psychodynamic, and focus instead on directly influencing behaviors, albeit through different means. Freeman and Eig address the patient's maladaptive cognitive schemas and the maladaptive core beliefs that make up those schemas using a variety of techniques These include Dysfunctional Thought Records and behavioral experiments aimed at generating experiences for the patient that challenge core beliefs and thereby alter schemas. Where there are specific skill deficits, these are addressed using more traditional behavior therapy techniques such as skills training and problem-solving training.

McCann and colleagues base their model in Dialectical Behavior Therapy developed by Linehan (1993). This model has strong connections to radical behaviorism, but also makes use of concepts from Buddhism and dialectical philosophy. In its practice, however, DBT as expounded by McCann and colleagues is more closely linked to behavioral analysis. Making extensive use of behavioral chain analysis, McCann and colleagues address the principal target behaviors in treatment through using these analyses to not only identify the components of the patient's problems, but also to identify intervention points and potential alternate responses to problematic situations.

Finally, one chapter, that by Ginsburg and colleagues, derives its theoretical focus from Rogerian therapy as incorporated into the Motivational Interviewing (MI) approach initially developed by Miller & Rollnick (2002) to work with substance abusers. MI relies almost exclusively on the therapeutic relationship developed between the client and therapist to reduce client ambivalence about change and enhance motivation to change behaviors that are selected by the client. Unlike the other approaches in this volume, MI does not take any specific position about the causes or methods of changing the behaviors that a client might select, but rather focuses on the power of an empathetic yet directive and reflective therapeutic relationship to reduce resistance and promote client-directed change.

These models represent pretty much the entire spectrum of types of psychotherapy as practiced in the early 21st century.

II. Essential Clinical Skills

The clinical skills that our authors point to as essential are surprisingly consistent across approaches. Essential skills cited in one fashion or another by all authors included ability to establish a working therapeutic relationship in which both empathy and objective feedback about the patient's behaviors was possible. Other essential clinical skills mentioned included flexibility, an ability to remain neutral and nonjudgmental in the face of patient provocativeness, skill in implementing the particular model adopted, and an ability to recognize and respond to countertransference that might arise.

McCann and colleagues focus most extensively on this last skill, advising the therapist working with patients with APD to engage in regular consultation with other similarly trained therapists to explore and recognize signs of potential therapist burn-out.

What is clear in these chapters is that virtually all of our authors view the establishment of a working therapeutic relationship and alliance with Frank as being at the core of successful treatment, regardless of the technical content of that treatment. The skills mentioned most often in this regard were an ability to both empathize and remain objective in response to Frank's behaviors and history. Given the provocativeness that many of our authors noted in Frank, it would seem that this aspect of treatment may be among the most challenging for therapists working with patients with APD.

III. Specific Questions

1.Therapeutic Goals.

In one form or another the most common therapeutic goal reported by our authors was the reduction of Frank's aggressive and destructive behavior. One set of authors (McCann et al.) saw this as a crucial task in conducting successful treatment with Frank, both from the standpoint of his outcomes and from the standpoint of therapist reactions to his potentially aggressive and threatening behavior.

A second common goal cited was that of teaching Frank more effective skills, including interpersonal problem-solving and social skills. Enhancing Frank's ability to relate appropriately to others was a therapeutic goal of five of the chapters.

Other goals focused on the establishment of a strong working relationship involving instilling in Frank a sense that therapy was a "safe" place where he could speak his mind without fear of sanction. In fact, for two of the approaches (Benveniste's psychodynamic approach and MI) the establishment of a working relationship was the primary goal cited.

The issue of who selects the goals seemed to divide our authors. Several chapters suggested specific goals that were largely determined by the therapist's assessment of Frank's problems, strengths, and weaknesses. Other authors specifically indicated that goals should be selected by Frank so as to be more relevant to, and motivating to, him. This stance toward goal setting appears to be in the interest of keeping Frank actively engaged in the therapeutic process through helping him develop a sense of personal ownership of the change process. This may be particularly important in coerced clients, such as Frank, where much resistance in treatment revolves around being "told" what to do!

2. Assessment/Further Information.

Not surprisingly, answers to the question regarding further information desired and assessments that might be done were quite variable. The authors of three of our chapters wanted some form of risk assessment, usually obtained through administration of the Psychopathy Checklist-Revised (Hare, 2003).

Nearly all of our authors wanted some form of personality and/or behavioral assessment, but the methods to be used in this assessment varied depending on whether the author's perspective was more psychodynamic or more behavioral. More psychodynamic authors wanted personality testing, most frequently the Rorschach, while more behaviorally oriented authors wanted specific behavioral analyses, sometimes obtained through use of theory-specific questionnaire measures such as the Young Schema Conceptualization Form (Young, 2002) or other theory-specific measures, such as Walters's Lifestyle Assessment of Criminal Thinking.

Surprisingly, only two authors wanted to interview collaterals, particularly Frank's wife and brother.

Other information that our authors cited as being useful were early recollections (Maniacci), evidence of pro-social thoughts and behaviors (Ginsburg et al.), and the client's agenda for being in treatment (Freeman & Eig).

3. Conceptualization of Personality, Behavior, Affective State, and Cognitions.

Answers to this question were among the most diverse we received from our authors.

Benveniste viewed Frank's behavior as having been shaped by two critical traumatic events: his mother's death and his subsequent ongoing abuse as a child. According to her conceptualization, these two events were instrumental in producing protective behavioral strategies and personality defenses that focused on self-protection and led to an inability to trust others enough to connect with them on a very basic level. This, in turn, led to his difficulties in relationships, particularly the lack of empathy for others that allowed Frank to be exploitive and manipulative.

Maniacci's formulation focuses on the short- and long-term goals or functions of Frank's behavior. Citing Frank's long-range goals of freedom, dominance, and control, Maniacci hypothesizes that these led to Frank's behavioral style of intimidation and a focus on pleasure seeking.

Dorr's conceptualization focuses on Millon's Polarities notion (Millon & Davis, 1996), postulating that Frank is weak on Preservation, Accommodation, and Nurturance, average on Enhancement, and strong on Individuating and Modifying. This leads to a strategy that focuses on reducing Frank's emphasis on self-gratification by reinforcing a sense of empathy and community. In the latter goal, Dorr agrees with Maniacci that helping Frank become better able to function in a community of others is a major issue to be addressed in treatment.

Walters views Frank's behaviors as due to an interaction of his environment, which reinforces specific maladaptive behaviors, and temperament. This interaction leads to maladaptive cognitions, emotions, and behaviors that facilitate Frank's criminal lifestyle. Changing these cognitions, emotions, and behaviors is the focus of treatment within the Lifestyle model.

Freeman and Eig conceptualize Frank's difficulties within the framework of cognitive behavior therapy. The focus here is on identifying problems and the psychological deficits that underlie them. Specifically, Freeman and Eig cite problems of poor self-control, thrill seeking, superficial and exploitive relationships, irresponsible behavior, authority problems, and Frank's tendency to blame others for his problems. These problems and deficits are all believed to stem from maladaptive cognitive schemas that influence how Frank perceives and relates to his work. These schemas are made up of core beliefs about the self, the world, and the future that need to be identified and modified in treatment.

McCann and colleagues are reluctant to speculate on a case conceptualization with extensive behavioral analyses that would identify both behaviors and the environmental contingencies that support them in a manner specific to Frank. Nonetheless, McCann and colleagues view Frank's central problem as aggression that is developed and maintained by a combination of biological predisposition and environmental contingencies supporting aggressive behavior. Also important in understanding Frank is an examination of his difficulties in emotional regulation, which is also the result of an interaction between biological factors (e.g., a tendency to be quickly aroused) and environmental contingencies that selectively reinforce behaviors arising from those biological factors.

Of the approaches represented, only the MI approach of Ginsburg and colleagues does not rely on a case conceptualization to understand Frank and guide his treatment. Rather, MI focuses on understanding the client in the context of the therapeutic relationship and in developing the patient's own view of his behavior and what should be the targets of change efforts, if any.

4. Potential Pitfalls.

The pitfalls identified by our authors fall into three broad types: therapist countertransference in response to what McCann and colleagues call "therapy-interfering behaviors," the resistance of patients with APD to change generally, and difficulties forming a strong working therapeutic relationship with Frank due to the first two factors. Several authors suggested caution with respect to the difficulty of the therapist maintaining a sense of objectivity and moral neutrality with respect to Frank's more florid behaviors, as well as a caution against being drawn into Frank's schemes as a result of his skillful manipulation of the therapist's empathy.

Also mentioned were therapeutic nihilism and the potential for a therapist to become discouraged by a lack of progress in Frank. This was linked by Benveniste with a caution against underestimating how difficult and complex a case Frank is, particularly with respect to the possibility that he is more psychopathic than he might appear.

Interestingly, only one set of authors, Ginsburg and colleagues, placed the focus of pitfalls and difficulties squarely on the therapist. Focusing on the implementation and spirit of MI, they cite such errors as engaging in a variety of traps that interfere with the therapeutic relationship (e.g., the therapist taking an "expert" stance toward Frank, or attempting to prematurely focus him on behavior change) as being major pitfalls to avoid. The ability to avoid these traps depends, they assert, to a large degree on how well-trained and experienced the therapist is.

5. Ultimate Level of Coping and Prognosis for Change.

Responses to this question reflected an extension of the traditional caution about hoping for too much change from patients with APD. Only Benveniste offered the possibility that Frank might change sufficiently so as to no longer meet diagnostic criteria for APD. This change would happen only if therapy was completed, and this would be likely to take 5–10 years, an unlikely prospect given the current emphasis on briefer treatments both by therapists and by third-party payers!

The rest of our authors had much more limited hopes for Frank. Completing his probation, reducing his tendencies toward impulsive and aggressive responses to problems, learning to adapt by focusing on the potential benefits of pro-social problem-solving, and a change in maladaptive schemas that lead to his problems, were all cited as possible changes. Largely absent was a prognosis of complete remission from APD.

One author, Maniacci, declined on theoretical grounds to speculate on prognosis at all, while the authors of the MI chapter focused their answer to this question on increased openness to exploring and committing to behavior changes selected by Frank himself.

6. Duration of Therapy.

Here the range of answers was quite large, ranging from 5–10 years of once or twice weekly individual sessions (Benveniste), to five hour-long individual sessions over the course of 5 weeks (Ginsburg et al.). Most responses clustered in a range of 12–24 months of weekly individual sessions, sometimes coupled with weekly group sessions. Only one author was unwilling to specify a possible duration of therapy (Dorr), largely due to the uncertain prognosis for change in patients with APD.

7. Specific/Special Techniques.

Here, again, the range of responses was large, with some form of confrontation being the most common technique cited. Confrontation was defined by all authors who suggested it as taking more the form of the therapist providing objective, non-judgmental feedback about Frank's behavior rather than the prescriptive, often aggressive, confrontation frequently associated with traditional substance-abuse treatments. All of our authors who suggested confrontation also indicated that it should be coupled with support and that it needed to occur only when the therapeutic alliance was reasonably well established. Dorr suggested that confrontation take the form of pointing out to Frank the harm his own behavior was causing him, thus capitalizing to a degree on his self-focused worldview.

Other techniques offered focused on intervening in and interrupting Frank's violent and aggressive behavior. Benveniste would do this by modeling appropriate behavior in session and reinforcing Frank for instances of less aggressive and self-aggrandizing behavior.

A number of authors focused on cognitive restructuring aimed at reducing criminogenic thought patterns and increasing Frank's ability to engage in effective problem-solving through skills training.

For Freeman and Eig, structuring sessions was a key technique. This would be done by use of agenda setting. They also suggest using behavioral experiments designed to assist Frank in questioning the validity of his core beliefs, thereby beginning the process of changing maladaptive schemas.

Ginsburg and colleagues focus on four specific techniques that are at the heart of MI: asking open-ended questions, affirming the client, reflective listening, and using summaries to help focus the client on his/her ambivalence. MI theory and research suggests that when these four techniques are regularly used by therapists, change occurs.

Finally, several of our authors cited some form of self-monitoring outside of sessions as an important component of Frank's therapy.

8. Special Cautions and Resistances.

The main cautions and potential resistances cited were Frank's tendency toward aggressive and disruptive behavior, and therapist countertransference. Frank, and other patients with APD, are easy to dislike, and their behaviors often evoke strong negative reactions in therapists. These reactions can get in the way of the formation of a strong therapeutic alliance, reduce therapist commitment to working with Frank, and, at their worst, lead to termination of treatment altogether either through Frank committing some violation of his probation and being incarcerated as a result, or through the therapist ending treatment due to lack of progress.

The upshot of this set of cautions and resistances was presented as the need to set clear and well-specified limits and establish clear personal and therapeutic boundaries with Frank. Failure to do so would likely lead, in the view of several authors, to behaviors that would produce negative countertransference or burnout in the therapist, and thus jeopardize treatment.

Only one set of authors, Ginsburg and colleagues, suggested no special cautions. In fact, within the framework of MI, resistance and possibly disruptive behaviors (stemming from ambivalence about change) are expected and viewed as a natural part of the change process.

9. Areas to Avoid.

There was surprising agreement among our authors in their response to this question. With the exception of avoiding exploration of past developmental issues and problems (Dorr), and avoiding prescription of a 12-step based approach to address Frank's drinking, everything about Frank's behavior, thinking, and feelings was considered grist for the therapeutic mill.

This said, Benveniste indicated that, while no topics were excluded from consideration *a priori,* the decision of whether or not to address specific topics is to some degree dependent on the phase of treatment. Thus, issues related to long-term personality changes should, according to Benveniste, be avoided in the early phase of therapy as being too threatening for Frank to address adequately.

10. Medication.

Here there was also surprising unanimity among our authors, with the caveat that even if medication would possibly be helpful as an adjunct to the work being done in psychotherapy, Frank might be very resistant to using medication at all.

Most frequently suggested medications were one or another of the SSRI antidepressants, mood stabilizers, and medications aimed specifically at Frank's drinking (either disulfiram or naltrexone). McCann and colleagues also suggested that the use of an atypical antipsychotic could be potentially beneficial, especially in containing Frank's tendency toward impulsive aggression.

These recommendations from our psychotherapy chapter authors are consistent with the more detailed account of the role of medication provided in the chapter by Freeman and Rathbun.

11. Patient Strengths.

While all of our authors saw strengths in Frank, a majority also cautioned that in patients with APD, some of these strengths could be a double-edged sword—used both in the service of positive changes as well as to thwart effective treatment.

Specifically, Frank was viewed by all as intelligent and by many as quite socially skilled and interpersonally perceptive. Whether these strengths were used positively or not would depend both on Frank's readiness to change, and on the therapist's skill in redirecting Frank's thinking and behavior in a more pro-social direction.

In addition to his intelligence and interpersonal skills, Frank was also perceived to be a leader, to have good survival skills, and to have a certain tenacity to his approach to problems that, if harnessed in the service of positive changes, could be very helpful to Frank in the long run.

Finally, the fact that Frank is relatively free of Axis-I pathology, with the exception of problems with alcohol, was seen by one author (Walters) as a strength that would simplify the process of therapy.

12. Limits and Boundaries.

The setting of clear boundaries and limits was considered by most of our authors to be a key to working effectively with Frank. Most often these limits and boundaries were aimed at protecting the therapist from negative reactions to Frank, from his exploitiveness and manipulativeness, and thereby enhancing the likelihood that negative countertransference would be avoided or minimized.

Clearly stating the ground rules of therapy, and both reinforcing them when Frank follows them and pointing out when he does not, were seen as very important in working with Frank.

McCann and colleagues focus almost exclusively on the therapist in their answer to this question, stating that attempting to establish boundaries with respect to Frank's behavior implies that he has no limits and requires external control. Rather, McCann and colleagues focus on the importance of the therapist identifying and communicating his/her own limits and boundaries clearly to the patient, and taking prompt action when those limits or boundaries have been breached.

For Ginsburg and colleagues, limits and boundaries are maintained through therapist adherence to the principles of MI. They believe it is important that the therapist be sensitive to areas that Frank does **not** want to bring up in sessions. When Frank has engaged in aggressive or manipulative behavior toward the therapist, these are dealt with through reflective listening and through a matter of fact and direct pointing out that limits and boundaries have been breached.

In addition to these suggestions, Dorr also suggests limiting unproductive storytelling in the session by refocusing the patient back onto the change issues at hand.

13. Involvement of Significant Others and Use of Homework.

All of our authors except Ginsburg and colleagues indicated that involving significant others (SOs), particularly some combination of Frank's wife, probation officer, and brother, and using homework would be useful with Frank. For Ginsburg and colleagues the use of homework and involvement of SOs is simply not a part of MI.

Other authors suggested a variety of types of homework assignments that might be helpful with Frank. Most common was written self-monitoring in the form of specifically designed formats such as the Daily Thought Record or Behavioral Chain Analyses, or simply journaling of Frank's thoughts and feelings. A particular focus of such homework was Frank's antisocial thinking.

Both Maniacci and Freeman and Eig suggest using homework that revolves around practicing problem solutions and behaviors generated in sessions in the outside world, and then reporting back the next session about the outcome of the new behavioral strategies.

14. Termination Issues/ Relapse Prevention.

All of our authors suggest that some form of relapse prevention plan be put in place at the end of Frank's treatment. Even our more psychodynamically oriented authors adopted a cognitive behavioral approach to relapse prevention planning. Developing specific "if A occurs, then I will do B" plans is seen as important by all of our authors.

One of our authors (Walters) suggested, in addition to a relapse prevention plan, scheduling several booster sessions to follow up on and reinforce new behaviors and problem-solving strategies learned in treatment.

A focus on relapse prevention in the context of "what's in it for Frank" was also considered important.

For the majority of our authors, the relapse prevention plan represented the basic task of termination. However, for Benveniste, termination was a much more complicated issue. Within her psychodynamic perspective, how the end of therapy would be handled depends on what led to its end. Termination due to problematic behaviors (e.g., a criminal act leading to re-arrest and/or incarceration) would be handled somewhat differently than termination arising as a result of a successful completion of the tasks of treatment. The latter would involve a review of the therapeutic journey and a reinforcing of the changes Frank had made, as well as generation of a relapse prevention plan. For non-successful endings, the therapist would send Frank a letter detailing her view of the difficulties he had experienced in therapy and any progress he had made with an invitation to revisit the therapy process at some point in the future.

15. Mechanisms of Change.

Our authors' answers to this question were again quite diverse.

For Benveniste and for Ginsburg and colleagues, the primary mechanism of change is the therapeutic relationship. For Benveniste, the specific aspects of the therapeutic relationship that effect change are the safety of the holding environment, work on ego functioning, teaching verbalization with appropriate affect, and therapist empathy.

For Ginsburg and colleagues the relationship forms the context in which the patient can enhance self-efficacy or hope that change is possible, repeatedly hear himself articulating the reasons for and against change, and hear his own arguments for change in the form of change talk.

For Dorr, the common factors present in all therapy: empathy, respect, and a sound therapeutic relationship in the context of expectancy for change, also operate in Frank's treatment. He also emphasizes the utility of Millon's model in understanding the patient and directing therapeutic interventions.

For Maniacci, change represents a realignment of Frank's priorities and the purposes of his behavior, rather than a reinvention or restructuring of his personality. This realignment occurs as a result of helping Frank recognize that many of his maladaptive behaviors can be used to further more positive ends.

For Walters, the mechanism of change is life itself. Change is viewed as a natural part of life, albeit one that patients frequently find anxiety-provoking. Anxiety-provoking though it is, change is impossible to avoid, according to Walters, and successful therapy involves helping clients recognize change as beneficial rather than frightening.

For the more behaviorally oriented of our authors, the primary mechanism of change is the learning of new, more adaptive thoughts and behaviors. For Freeman and Eig, the focus is more on changing thoughts, with those changing leading to changes in behavior, while for McCann and colleagues the primary mechanism is learning new skills, as well as reshaping environmental contingencies to reinforce their use, although restructuring of maladaptive cognitions also plays a role.

IV. Conclusion.

It seems clear that, despite significant theoretical differences in the rationale for their use, a number of common approaches emerge that cut across our authors' approaches to working with patients like Frank. First is the crucial importance of establishing a working therapeutic alliance based on empathy, respect for Frank as a person, and an ability on the part of the therapist to give Frank objective, non-judgmental feedback about his behavior.

All of our authors also place great emphasis on helping Frank learn new ways of thinking and behaving that bring him closer to others, rather than increasing the gulf between Frank and the rest of the world. Thus, there is an emphasis on helping Frank begin to see himself as a member of a larger community of others whose feelings are also important, and with whom he can choose to relate either in a productive, collaborative way or as an adversary.

Skills training, especially with respect to relapse prevention, forms a part of all of our authors' models, with the sole exception the more limited (at least in terms of immediate therapeutic goals) MI.

Finally, our authors largely agree on the importance of structure, limits, and boundaries as critical to successful therapy with Frank.

These views largely converge with research on the treatment of criminal offenders, a group that has a large percentage of members who qualify for a diagnosis of APD. This research (Ross & Gendreau, 1980) suggests that treatments that are highly structured, with clear boundaries and limits, delivered in a respectful and empathetic but firm manner, and which incorporate behavioral skills and problem-solving training, have the best record of successful outcomes. What is now needed, in our view, is research examining the importance of these central variables in working with both criminal and non-criminal patients with APD. It is our hope that this book will provide an impetus for researchers to begin exploring this issue more widely. We also hope that this book will help in dispelling the notion that persons with APD are "untreatable," and encourage more psychotherapists to consider including these individuals in their practices.

REFERENCES

Hare, R.D. (2003). *Hare PCL-R technical manual* (2nd ed.). N. Tonawonda, NY: MHS.

Linehan, M.M. (1993). *Cognitive-behavioral treatment of borderline personality disorders.* New York: Guilford.

Miller, W.R., & Rollnick, S. (2002). *Motivational interviewing: Preparing people for change* (2nd ed.). New York: Guilford.

Millon, T., & Davis, R.D. (Eds.). (1996). *Disorders of personality: DSM-IV and beyond* (2nd ed.). New York: John Wiley.

Ross, R.R., & Gendreau, P. (1980). *Effective correctional treatment.* Scarborough, Ontario, Canada: Butterworth.

Young, J.E. (2002). Schema-focused therapy for personality disorders. In G. Simos (Ed.), *Cognitive behaviour therapy: A guide for the practicing clinician* (pp. 201–222). New York: Taylor & Francis.

Index